This book belongs to: _____

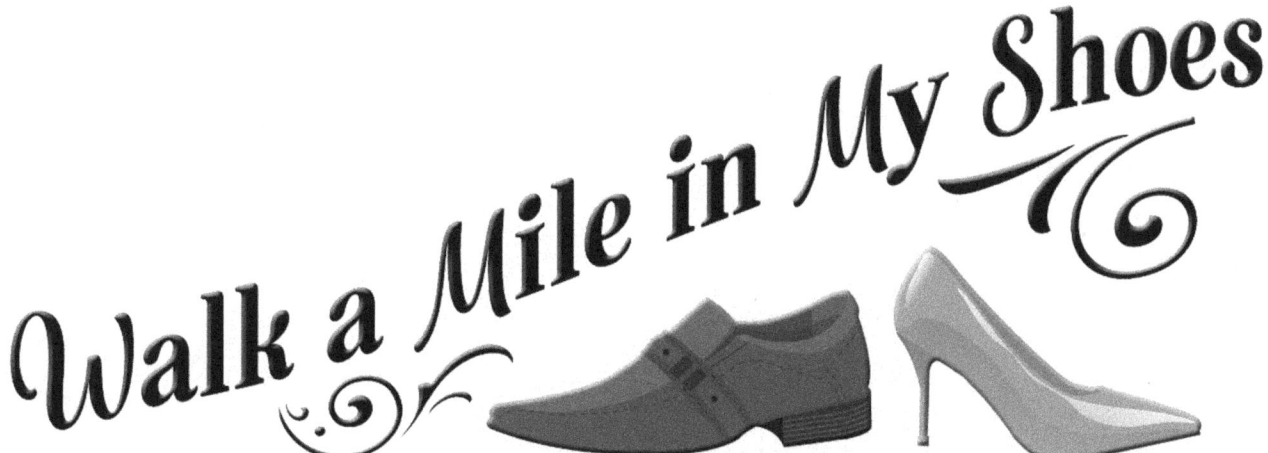

A Solution-Oriented Training for Employees of a Chronic Pain Practice

Dedication

For Dr. Christian "Kris" Obah, M.D.

Thank you for your kinder, gentler manner, and for genuinely caring about your patients. Thank you, most of all, for treating me with humanity— not an atypical 'migraine', but a bright, capable *person* who suffers from an atypical migraine.

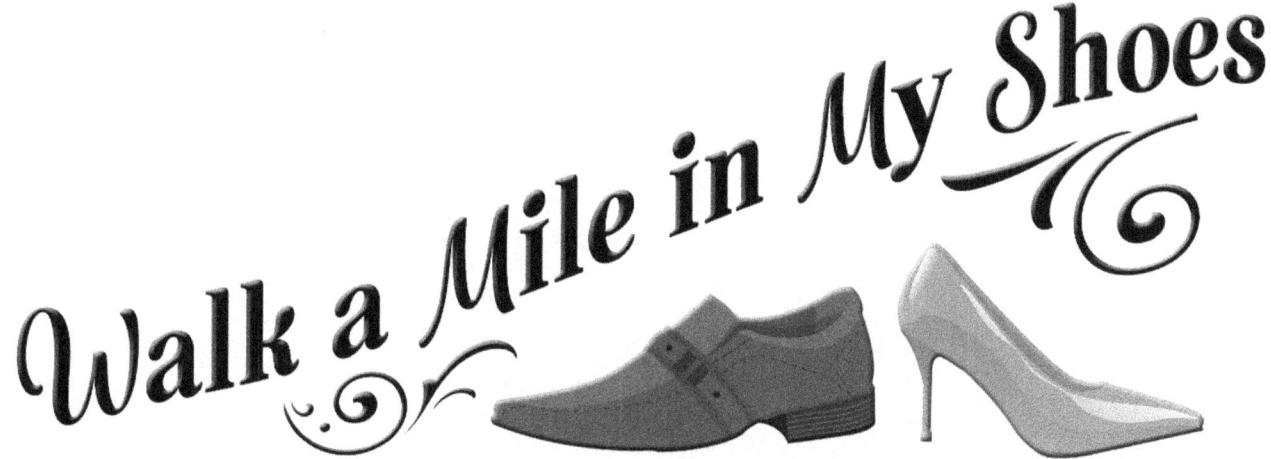

A Solution-Oriented Training for Employees of a Chronic Pain Practice

USA TODAY Bestselling Author

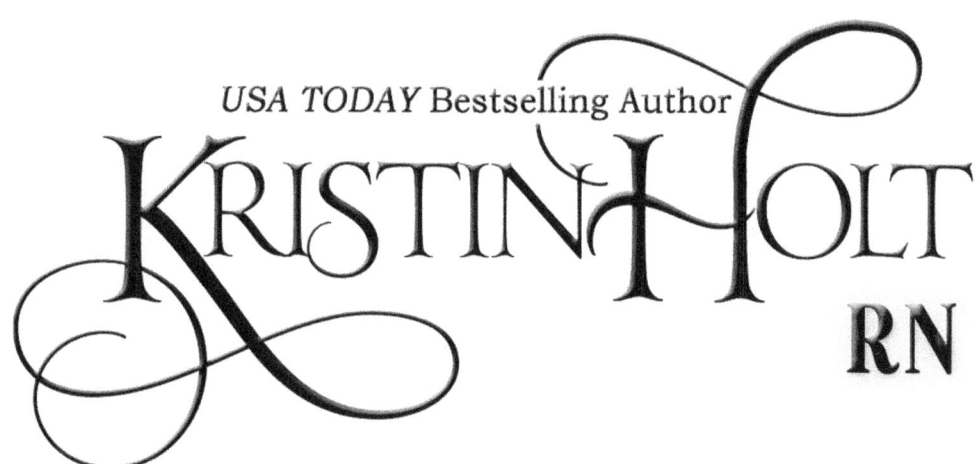

Kristin Holt, RN

A WALK IN MY SHOES: A SOLUTION-ORIENTED TRAINING FOR EMPLOYEES OF A CHRONIC PAIN PRACTICE

Copyright © 2019 by Kristin Holt LC

All rights reserved. Except as permitted under the U.S. Copyright Act of 1976, no part of this publication may be reproduced, distributed, or transmitted in any form or by any means now known or hereafter invented, or stored in a database or retrieval system, without the prior written permission of the publisher, Kristin Holt.

Cover Art by Kristin Holt
Cover Design by Kristin Holt
Interior Design by Kristin Holt

Photographs and vectors used with a paid premium subscription to Freepik.com (with minor exceptions)
Approximately five unique images used with a paid subscription to CreativeFabrica.com
Pain Scale and Satisfaction Scale, freeware
Family photograph Kylee Ann Studios, used with permission
Word Art © 2019 by Kristin Holt LC

First Edition
First Printing, 2019

ISBN: 978-1-63438-043-0
Published by Kristin Holt LC
www.KristinHolt.com

Table of Contents
Walk a Mile in My Shoes

Description	6
Chapter One: 1/10 mile: Why I'm Worth Listening To	7
Chapter Two: 2/10 mile: Chronic Pain, Stats and Reality	11
Chapter Three: 3/10 mile: Customer-Related Challenges I Face Daily	15
Chapter Four: 4/10 mile: What is Your *Greatest* Challenge?	17
Chapter Five: 5/10 mile: Angry Patients	21
Chapter Six: 6/10 mile: Anxious Patients	27
Chapter Seven: 7/10 mile: Need a Break? Step away. Breathe.	35
Compassion Fatigue	36
Chapter Eight: 8/10 mile: Three Simple Tools	37
Leave Your Stuff at the Door	40
Empathy / Sympathy / Compassion	47
Kindness	55
Chapter Nine: 9/10 mile: Commitment to Try the Tools	65
Chapter Ten: 10/10 mile: Important Questions	67
Thank You	71
Training Evaluation	75
Appendix A: Twenty-four Pain Lessons	77

Description

Of all personnel in all medical offices, I submit that employees in Pain Management practices (or clinics) have among the most difficult, challenging, and draining work experiences. Why? Because *every single patient* is in pain. And grumpy. Short-tempered, too.

Is it possible to safeguard my emotional reserves *and* demonstrate superior customer service? YES!

Can I go home at the end of the day overflowing with optimism and pleasure instead of exhausted and wrung dry? YES!

Walk a Mile in My Shoes identifies your greatest workplace challenges. Three actionable Tools *reduce your burdens, elevate your mood, increase job satisfaction*, and *reduce the "chafe"* of those workplace challenges. Inside, you'll find the right words, the simplest of methods, and instead of giving and giving until you're threadbare, learn to fill your own well even as you excel in your role with patients.

This manual was developed to accompany a one-hour live training presentation by the same name. This book might substitute for the group training, as it contains most of the presentation's content, and in many sections, includes much more: video links, additional insights, supportive articles, quotes, room for personal lists, self-assessment questions, and space to write down epiphanies and discoveries.

<u>Are you a Pain Management Office administrator planning to train staff members?</u> With your purchase of this workbook for each participant, and upon email request, the author will provide via email the PowerPoint presentation and training notes, as is, and free of charge.

Kristin Holt, RN, brings "three sets of shoes" to the "shoe swap" of *Walk A Mile in My Shoes*. The point where these three shoes—or three defining experiences in her life—create ideal credibility. Her nursing specialty was Labor and Delivery, where she experienced firsthand what pain does to nice and gracious people. Then Pain knocked on her door, became an unwanted house guest, and two decades later, Kristin knows what it's like to live with severe chronic pain. As a Weight Watchers™ Receptionist, Leader, and ultimately, Territory Manager, superb customer care became paramount as Kristin trained hundreds of employees in customer care, and coached them to peak performance.

Chapter One
1/10 mile: Why I'm Worth Listening To

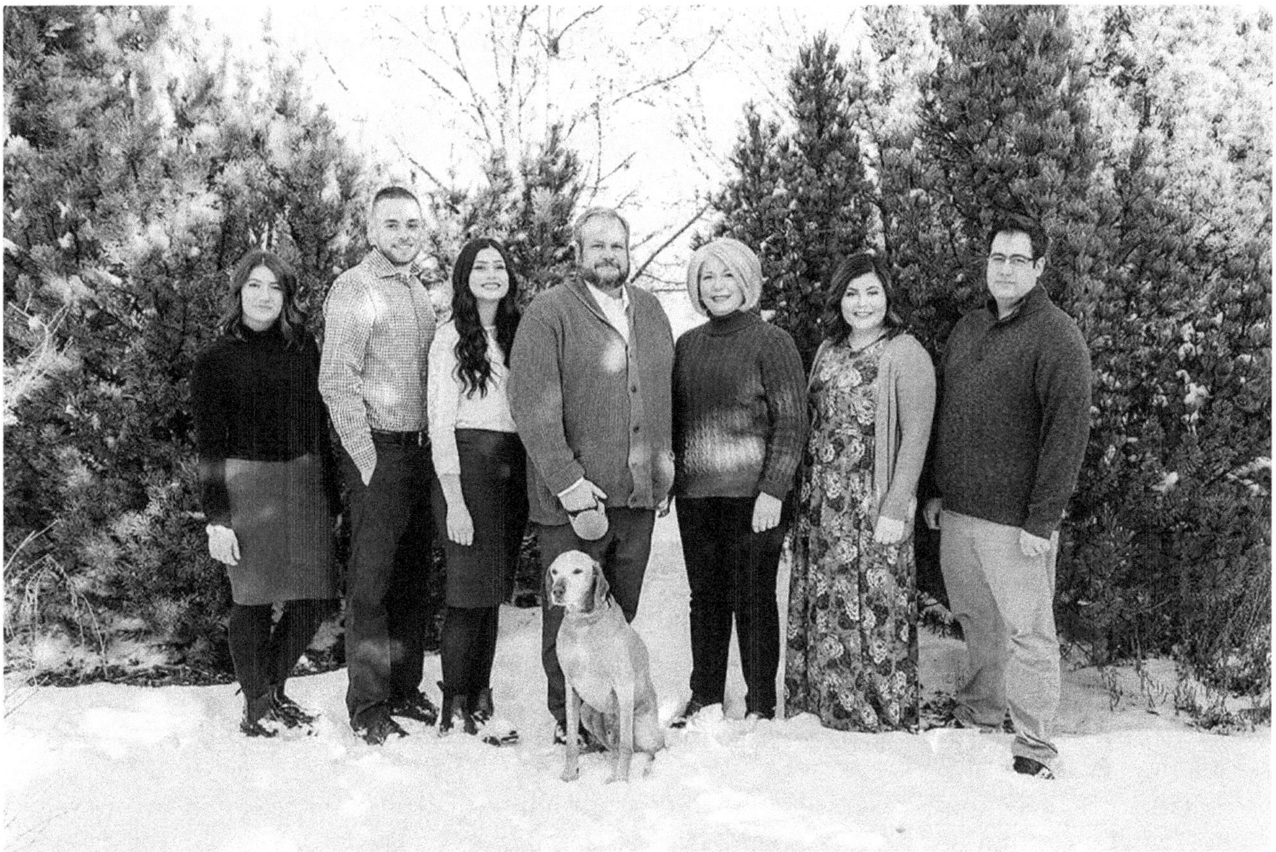

Kristin Holt and Family

Allow me to introduce myself. My name is Kristin Holt. I'm a Registered Nurse with a specialty in Labor and Delivery and a Certified Childbirth Educator. I married within a few years of completing my university education, and my husband and I will celebrate our thirty-first anniversary this spring. We're the proud parents of four adult children (and one son-in-law); our children have excelled in their education. Much like their father (with a Masters Degree in Engineering), our offspring LOVE math. Our son is an IT Specialist, our eldest daughter a math teacher at a high school, our middle daughter is Masters Prepared Bio-Statistician, her husband a Human Resources Specialist, and our youngest daughter is an upperclassman studying to become an actuary for insurance companies (another variation of statistics).

I was young, well-educated, competent, confident, and in charge.

I had friends—lots of them.

I made dinner every single night for our growing children (and my husband). I read and sewed and cross-stitched for enjoyment. I taught myself through a great deal of study and reading how to bottle fruit and to knit sweaters.

Life was good.

I may have had a few more headaches than my friends in high school, and by college, I had headaches a couple times a week. Often, annoying, but no big deal.

By the time our fourth child was born, I had headaches almost every day; by the time she was five, I was significantly impacted by headaches that have since become "brain fire". After all, 'headache' is a mild term and won't take into account the enormous pressure of a tank parked on my skull, the white-hot skewer poking through my skull, and the 'fact' that my brain is ON FIRE.

Through the early years, I managed to work full time as a Receptionist, Leader, and ultimately a Territory Manager for Weight Watchers. I led Weight Watchers meetings weekly. I interviewed and hired. I trained new employees. I conducted various trainings on a frequent basis. I drove a company car and had more than full-time responsibilities to the company.

The Brain Fire became so severe I was ultimately unable to continue. I simply couldn't work for someone else any longer. I needed far too many hours in bed. The pain had taken on a life of its own and I could no longer manage well enough to work long days, drive hundreds of miles each week, and burn the candle at both ends.

For several years, I managed to work for myself, picking up a hobby from many years ago when my children were small. I've written more than 20 titles (novels, novellas, and short stories), and have had the wonderful experience of a title landing on the *USA Today* Bestsellers List.

Through these many years, I've been in so much pain I can't write. I can't work, can't sleep, can't attend my family's social events, I can't exercise, can't go to the movies. Microphones and organs and all forms of amplified sound are excruciating. I've lost more than 50% of my daylight hours to severe chronic pain. I need to earn an income, and can't.

I went from interacting with many people every single day to speaking pretty much only with immediate family members– and if I'm lucky, one other person per day.

I am Qualified to Address this Subject

I know the life of a busy, full-time-and-more employed wife/mother because I've lived it.

I know the insanity of a busy Labor & Delivery job because I've lived it.

I know the desperation and anxiety of severe chronic pain because I've lived it.

I spent a decade immersed in Customer Service, training and coaching others.

Let's walk in one another's shoes as we explore the challenges of chronic pain—for patients *and* for employees of a chronic pain clinic. We'll begin with the reason we're here. Patients in pain.

A Patient in Pain

Do you *know what it's like* to be in *prolonged* pain?

I'll emphasize again; do you *know*? Do you?

Have you had a bout with kidney stones? Or a gallbladder episode that ended up in the O.R.?

Have you given birth? Whether hours and hours of labor or by Cesarean Section it matters not. Both types of deliveries bring intimacy with pain.

Knee surgery? Hip replacement surgery? Breast reduction or enlargement surgery?

Have you injured your back and spent weeks nearly immobile?

Experienced dental pain that interrupted your life with every snack and every sip?

Have you survived a car accident?

This list is far from complete. *Far from it*. If you've known any one of these things, and several hundred thousand beyond its finite number, you have my sincere sympathies. Welcome to the exclusive club neither of us wants.

My Experiences with Pain

_____

_____

_____

_____

_____

Do I Feel Compassion for Those in Pain?
Really? Deep-down?

___

___

___

___

Twenty-four Pain Lessons
See Appendix A containing twenty-four Pain Lessons.

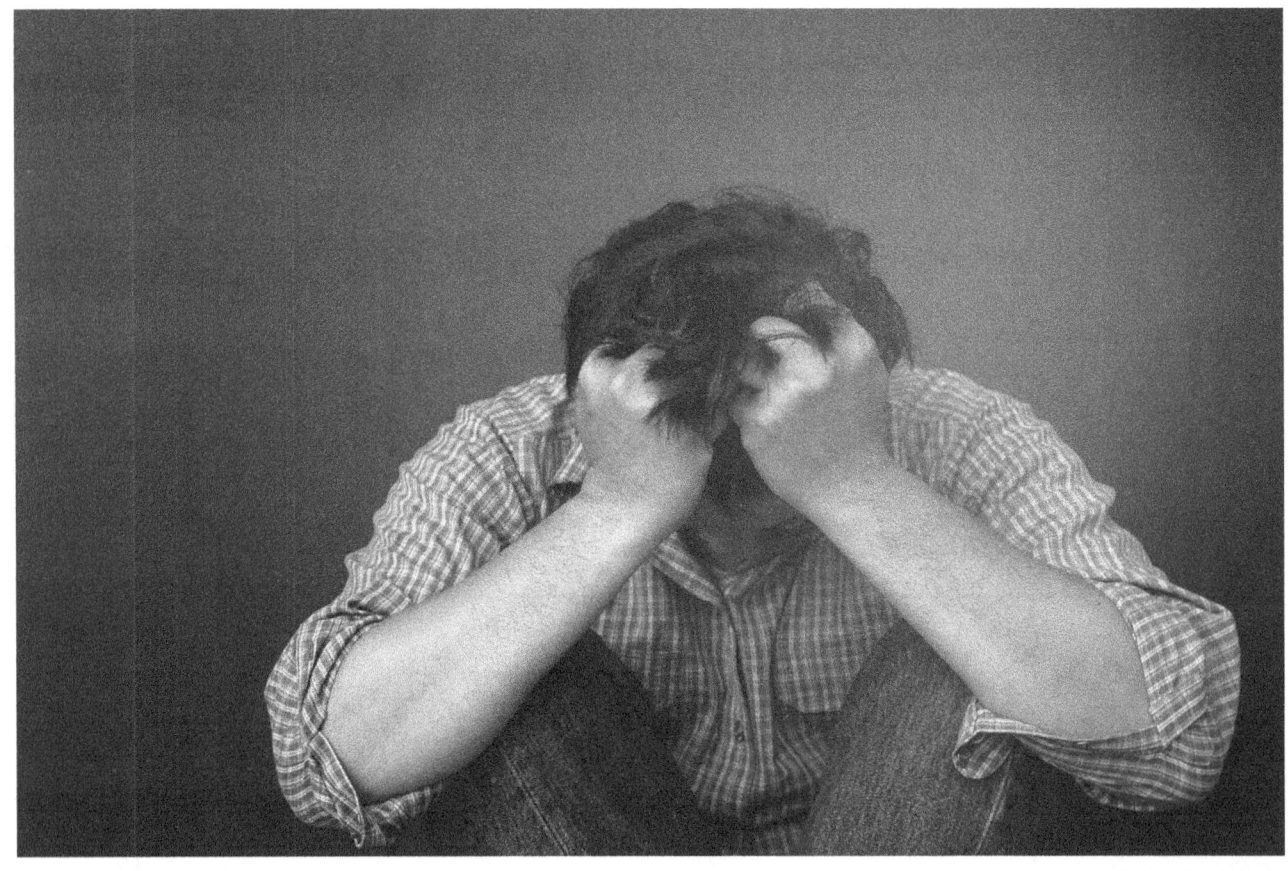

Chapter Two
2/10 mile: Chronic Pain, Stats and Reality

Chronic Pain-- A club no one wants to join

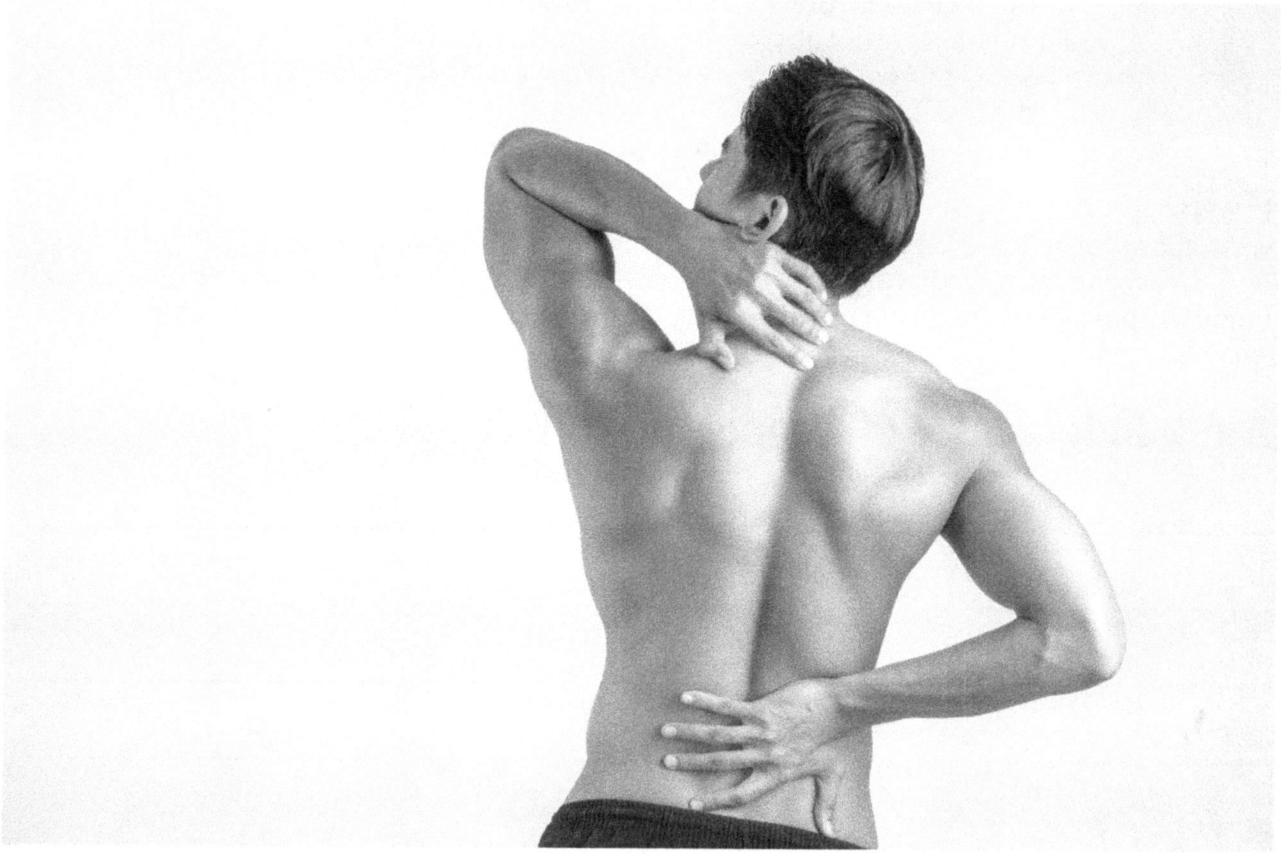

Statistics

According to *Journal of Pain*[1], a cross-sectional, Internet-based survey (with a nationally representative sample of adults in the United States) determined **nearly 31% suffer from chronic pain**[2]. Prevalence was higher among females than males and increased as the patients age. Chronic low back pain was the number one most frequent complaint.

A variety of sources claim the number of Americans is significantly higher or lower than this. I'd have to ask my statistician daughter about that. I'm guessing the answer isn't so simple.

A Glimpse Inside

" "Low Back Pain is the leading cause of disability in the world.

80% of U.S. adults will experience back pain at some point in their lives.

Back pain is one of the most common reasons for missed work, and the second-leading cause for doctor's visits.

Pain is a significant public health problem, costing society at least $560 to $635 billion annually (that's $2K for EVERYONE living the U.S.)

Currently, over 4,000 doctors practice Pain Management."[3]

Pain

Remember, once upon a time, when pain meant something was wrong?

Everyone involved with chronic pain—whether the patient, researcher, family member, physician, medical support staff—knows that the rules aren't so simple.

Am I Judgmental of People in Pain? Explain.

_____

_____

_____

_____

---

[1] *Journal of Pain*, November 2010, Volume 11, Issue 11

[2] chronic, recurrent, long-lasting pain with a duration of at least 6 months

[3] https://paindoctor.com/resources/chronic-pain-statistics/

What does lack of judgment look like?

_____
_____
_____
_____
_____
_____

Pain is a short-term symptom of an easily corrected situation.

Usually.

Fill in the blanks:

I think that the people who are patients at our pain management office/clinic are _____ and need _____ and _____. I've found that staff members with personality traits like _____ and _____ and _____ enjoy the work more than those who don't.

The reason we lose employees to other jobs is because _____.

Those who stay _____.

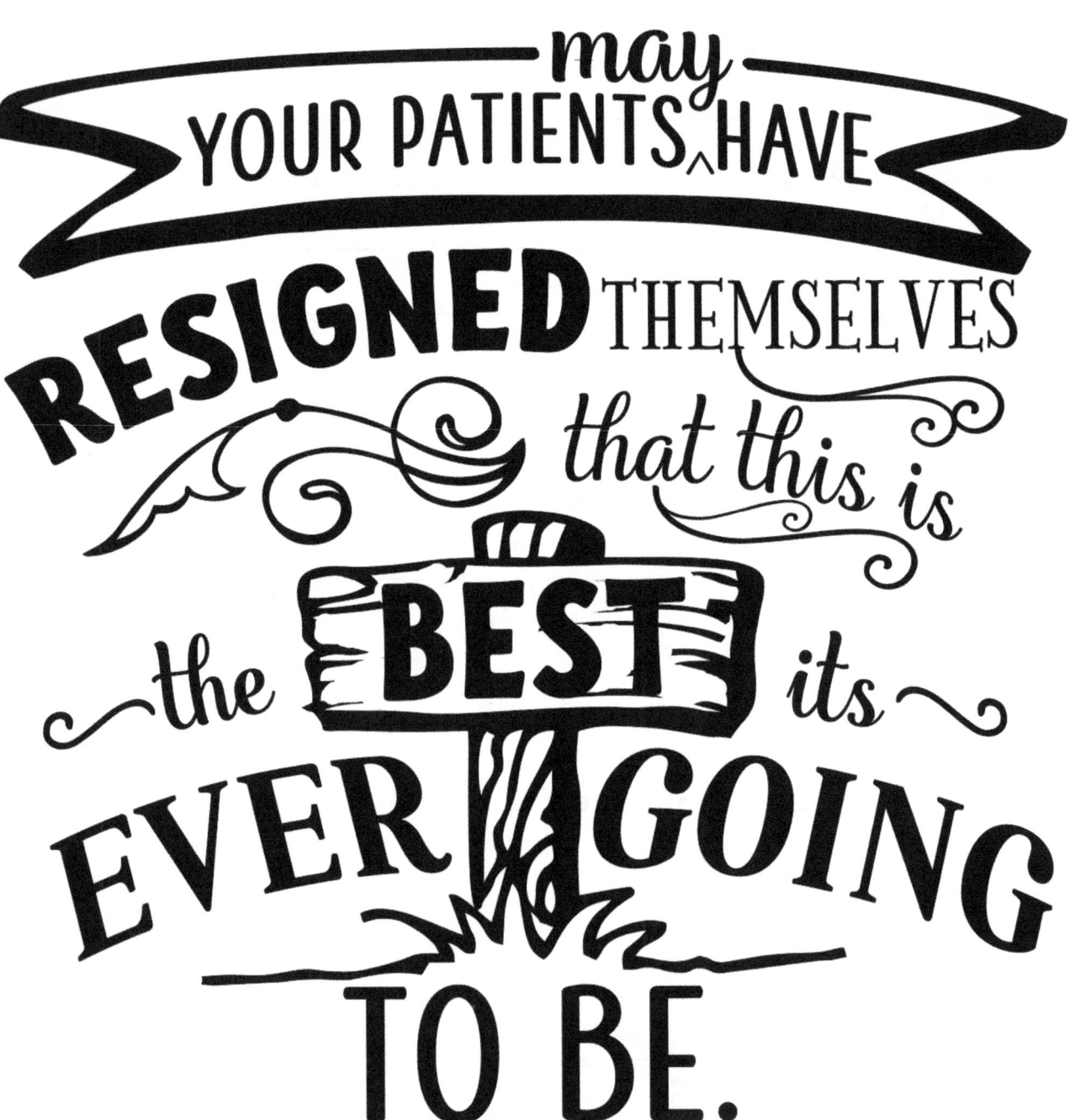

Chapter Three
3/10 mile: Customer-Realted Challenges I Face Daily

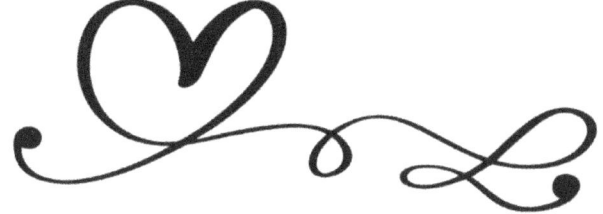

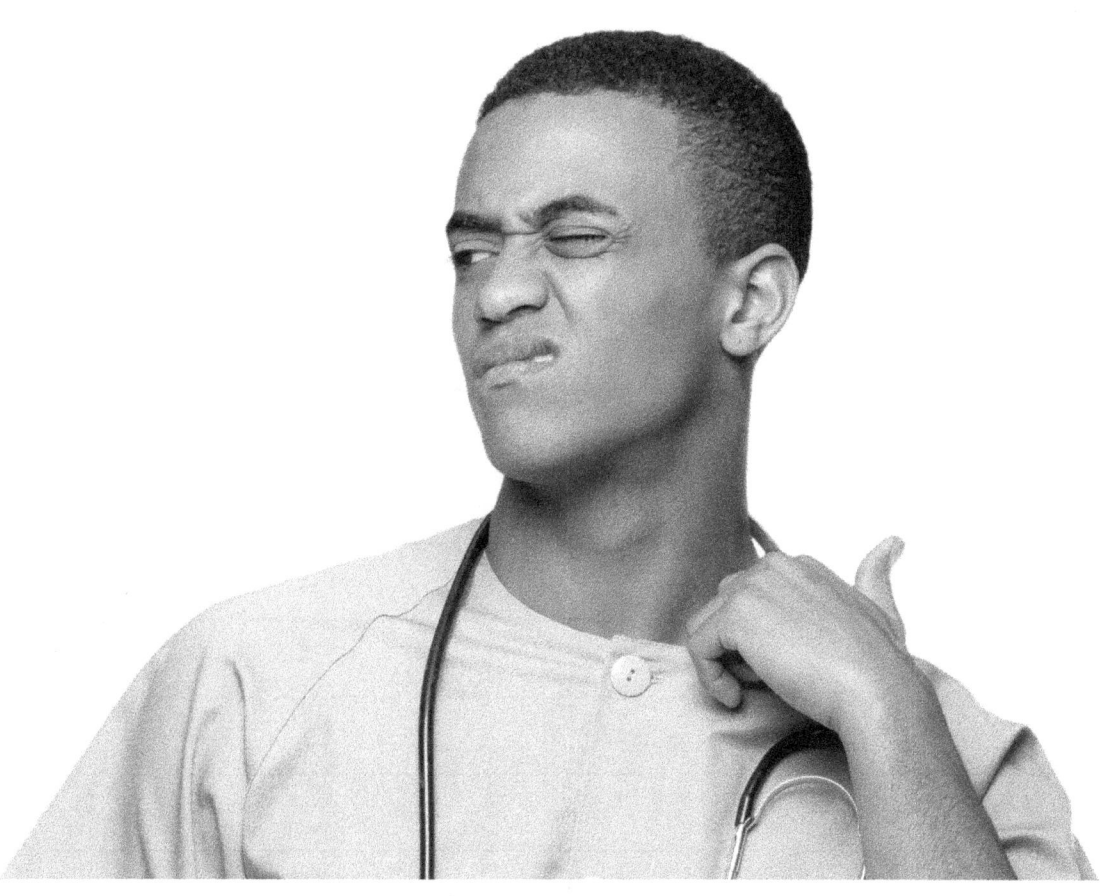

I work in a high-stress, high-demand industry.

Customer-Related Challenges I Face Daily Because I Work with Chronic Pain Patients.

<u>This list is PRIVATE</u>.

Jot down everything you can think of—every bit of friction, conflict, and "I hate this part of my job." Don't think too hard—you have only 60 seconds.

_____

_____

_____

_____

_____

_____

_____

_____

_____

_____

_____

_____

_____

_____

Chapter Four
4/10 mile: My Greatest Customer-Related Challenge at Work

Look at your list. Are the most important issues represented?
Which one or two or even three saps **your personal energy and wears you thin?** Got them? Star the biggies.
Live training participants-- are you ready to share? *Answers will be posted*—but all *contributors will remain anonymous*. No names will be displayed or disclosed.

Jot your top answers here, if you wish

_____
_____
_____
_____
_____
_____
_____
_____

Truth: **People in pain aren't always very nice.**

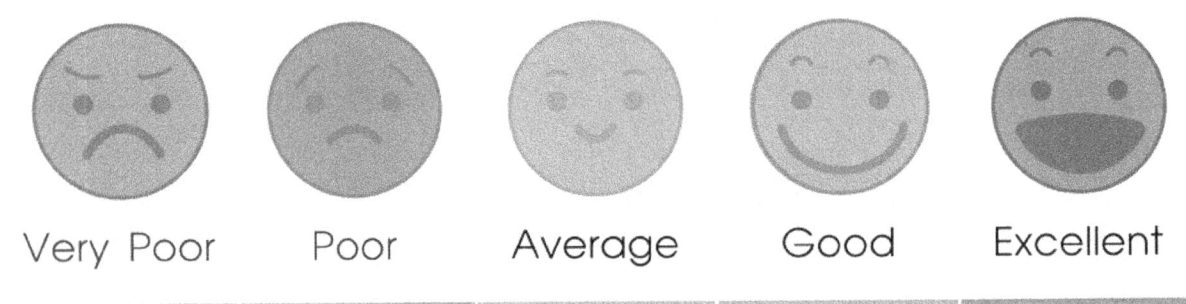

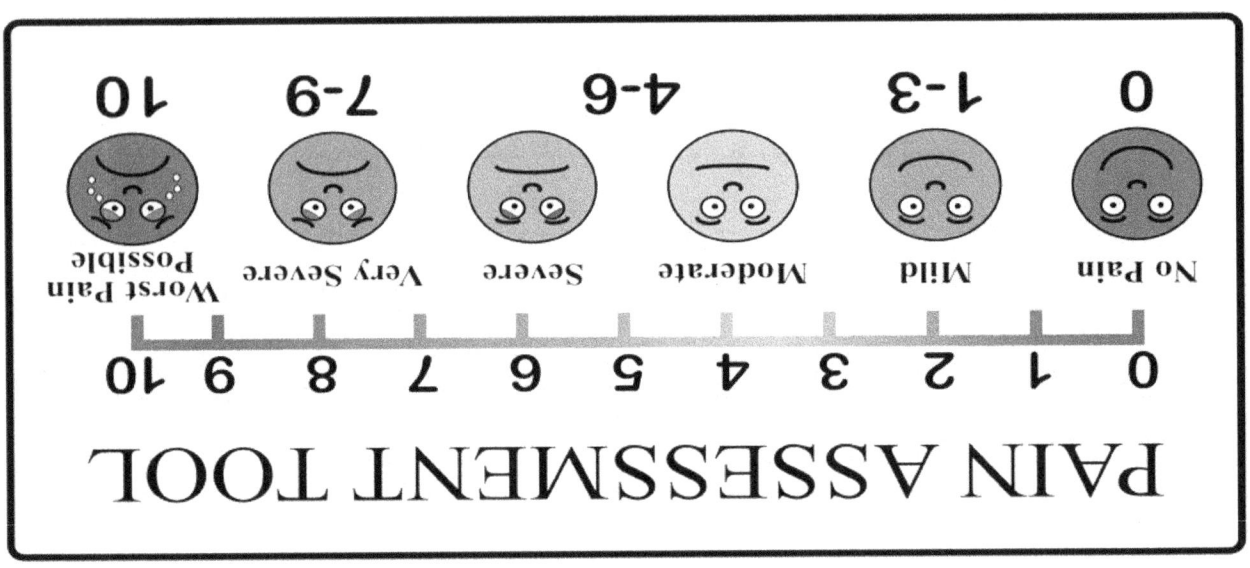

What do you enjoy most about your work in pain management?

___

Why do you suppose this is?

___

Notes:

Chapter Five
5/10 mile: Angry Patients

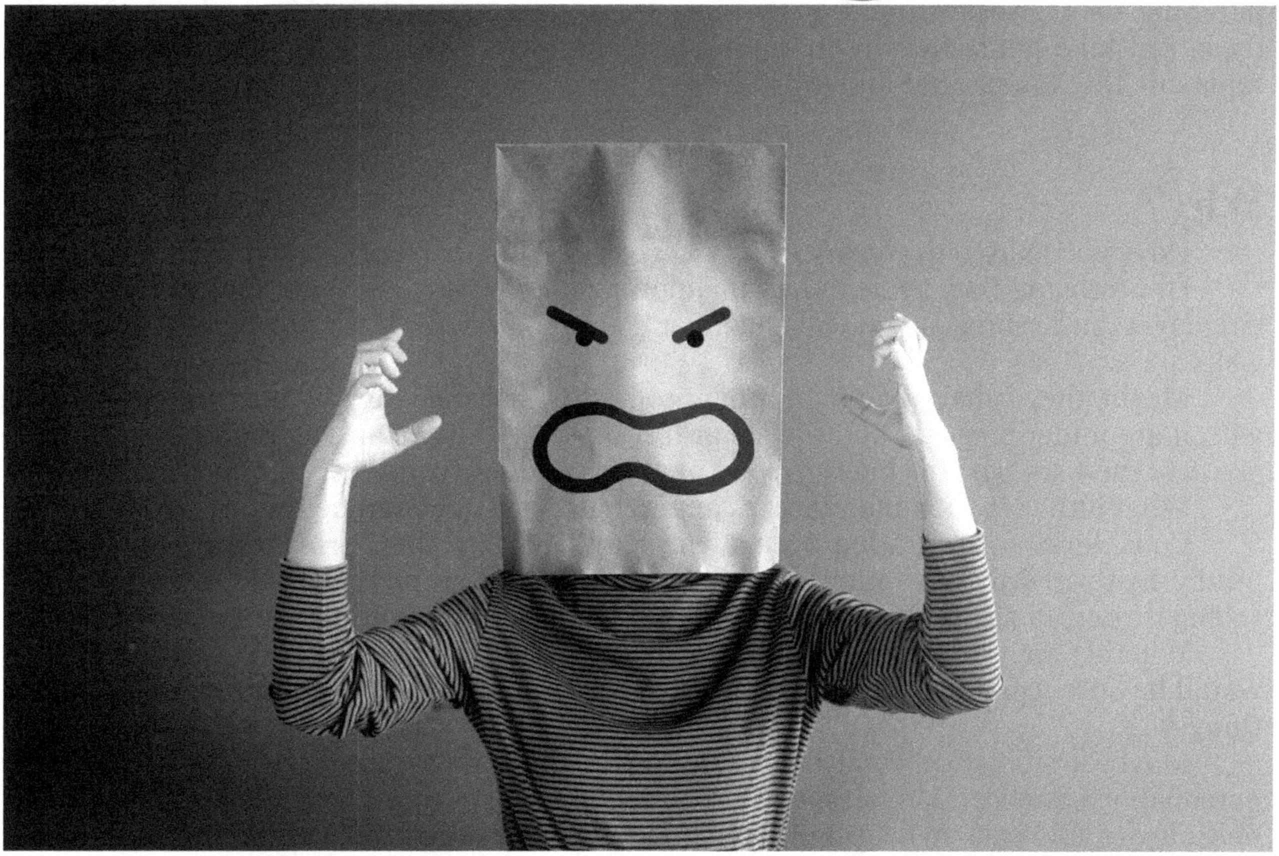

SEEK FIRST TO UNDERSTAND.
THEN TO BE UNDERSTOOD.
~ Steven Covey

The Angry Patient

Oh, boy. Lots of fun.

According to some circles, angry patients are the dominant category of "problem" patients, a.k.a. <u>Dweebus Patients</u> according to my brother-in-law, a family physician.

Angry patients/clients raise their voices. They yell and scold and call names and heap accusations upon accusations. Body posture exudes threat.

I've discovered it matters little (at least to me) whether this Angry Patient Attack is over the phone or in person. The visceral reaction is the same. The pulse spikes. Defense mechanisms flash to high alert, large muscle groups tighten, and the voice shakes. Oh, and perspiration. Lots of perspiration. Heartbeats pound in the ears, but adrenaline is pumping on high speed, and everything, every threat, registers. Visceral reactions like these can take hours to fully dissipate. Usually longer, as our minds tend to ruminate, replaying the trauma over and over.

Yuck.

Why?

Have you paused to consider WHY *Dweebus Patients* bite the hands that feed them?

Honestly, do they believe that abandoning all courtesy, spewing foul words in three languages, and yelling at you will engender your good favor? Make you want to treat them well?

Maybe they behave badly and inappropriately because the volatile, roiling emotions within are under pressure and the steam-release valve allows an anger eruption. Chances are they can't see past the big red cloud of anger to identify the real emotion inside.

What if the emotion manifests as anger, but that's not what lies beneath it all?

Consider how frustration over a lengthy wait to see their provider might flash past mildly frustrated to screaming mad with accelerants like physical pain, emotional pain (going through a divorce), and anxiety (the kid wants to live with the other parent).

Whether we want to or not, we grieve the loss of the life that we'd always imagined would be ours... that end of the pathway we'd chosen for ourselves. Grief Therapy is a real thing.

Maybe a statistical analysis would prove me wrong, but here's the truth of my personal experience. I saw specialist after specialist: internist, neurologist, another neurologist, and back to a trusted family doctor whose diagnostic abilities engendered my trust. I think most patients suffer for a good, long while before they ever arrive at a pain management clinic as a first-time patient. Chances are they waited a month for an appointment with their family medicine doctor only to be told that pain management is a specialty and they'll need to see someone in that field. Cue more waiting.

Your patients are unique. No doubt about that. We all know that a treatment that worked for Mr. A's lower back pain did squat for Mr. B's lower back pain. When it comes to the impact of pain upon our manners and tolerance and patience, another wide range. I'd hope many of us still behave like ladies and gentlemen.

Many are short-tempered, nasty, critical, and volatile.

I hope that by now, you can sense what putting on the shoes of a chronic pain sufferer and walking around the block over and over would be like.

Imagine yourself in a situation where you're in pain. Noticeable, big pain. Pain that's white-hot and continuous. Oh, and it's likely going to last the rest of your lifetime.

Add to this that you've been looking for answers and solutions, and this has been going on for *years*.

You had plans. Big plans. Perhaps you weren't done with your education. Or you'd only begun dating a fabulous person...

And sleep last night was a joke. Not a chance of sleeping, much less sleeping well.

The pain meds help, but only a little.

All of this, combined with waning hope, can make folks unbelievably cranky.

How?

How to handle an altercation with an angry patient...

You've probably attended three-day conferences dedicated to the subject.

You've learned to effectively shut down combative clients, either at such trainings or by your own experience, including watching someone else manage a combative client superbly or miserably.

If the anger is over a billing error, and the client is willing to have a dialog and discover the solution, then that's a straightforward solution. We could create a list with a thousand situations that might spark a confrontation in the pain clinic. Some are relatively straightforward and others are ugly with limited solutions.

No matter what those underlying reasons for conflict are, a simple list of Best Practices will help to diffuse the client's anger and facilitate open communication.

Best Practices

1. **LISTEN**; the person desperately wants to feel *heard*.
    a. LISTEN without forming your reply, or without racing ahead to find a solution. Just LISTEN.
    b. Set aside anything else – undivided attention will ensure the patient sees you're trying.
    c. Open body language
    d. Eye contact
    e. Encourage the person to continue, and share the rest of the circumstances or events.
2. **Express a Desire to Help**
    a. "I want to help."
    b. "Help me to understand so I can help make things right."
    c. "I'll take this information to our office administrator."
    d. When appropriate (likely the majority of the time), bring the office administrator into the conversation.

3. **Acknowledge, validate, rephrase**
    a. "I see you're upset." (this gives the person a chance to either A) feel heard or B) disagree and tell you how they do feel)
    b. "I'd be unhappy too."
    c. "I wouldn't like that either."
    d. "You're saying you (the phrase the person used)?"
    e. "Thank you for telling me about this."
4. **Apologize** (without admitting fault)
    a. "I'm so sorry this has happened."
    b. Never throw someone else under the bus. Never hint that a coworker has done something wrong or against policy. "We ARE they."
    c. You can speak generally as "we" to apologize and encourage. "We want you to feel comfortable here. We're sorry the TV is too loud. I've turned it down."
5. **ASK**; ask the patient how he/she thinks the matter would be best resolved.[4]
    a. For example, you could say: *"I understand you're angry about XYZ. What can I do to help you feel understood?"* [5]
    b. Listen far more than you speak (at least until the entire explanation has been heard), but while you listen make sure you use Active Listening skills: nod to encourage continuation, use a hand gesture to signal "keep going," or a brief word or phrase, e.g., "What happened then?" or "Say more."

Defense Against an Attack

Once in a blue moon, a client's anger goes well beyond the conversation stage. Or perhaps you don't have a counter between you and the verbally abusive person.

You've likely attended day-long events about dealing with combative patients or those who are out of control or beyond reason.

One such strategy is to stand up for yourself. Interrupt if you have to. Talk loudly, decisively, infusing as much authority into your voice as possible. "I'm going to end this conversation right now." In most cases, you'll have the person(s) attention. The power will shift back to you.

This "counter-attack" should be used only as a means of last resort (IMHO), as it tends to announce, literally, "we're done talking", and will kill the possibility until one or both parties calm down (and perhaps long thereafter).

---

[4] https://www.patientpop.com/blog/running-a-practice/patient-experience/5-strategies-for-dealing-with-problem-patients-and-when-you-should-let-them-go/

[5] https://www.patientpop.com/blog/running-a-practice/patient-experience/5-strategies-for-dealing-with-problem-patients-and-when-you-should-let-them-go/

Excellent Resources

Scan QR code OR type the following link into your search window:

http://www.hpso.com/risk-education/individuals/articles/Handling-the-Angry-Patient

Scan QR code or type the following into your search window:
https://www.thehappymd.com/blog/bid/290399/doctor-patient-communication-the-universal-upset-patient-protocol
Don't miss the video! It's helpful.

Scan QR code or type the following into your search window:

https://www.nursebuff.com/how-to-handle-angry-patients-and-families/

Scan QR code or type the following into your search window:

https://journals.lww.com/nursing/FullText/2008/05000/Dealing_with_an_angry_patient.32.aspx

An example of an upset, angry client ~ and the situation was handled very well

_____
_____
_____
_____
_____
_____
_____
_____
_____
_____
_____

If necessary, recall an example where things were handled poorly. What did you learn?

I THRIVE IN PAIN MANAGEMENT. What's your Superpower?

Chapter Six
6/10 mile: Anxious Patients

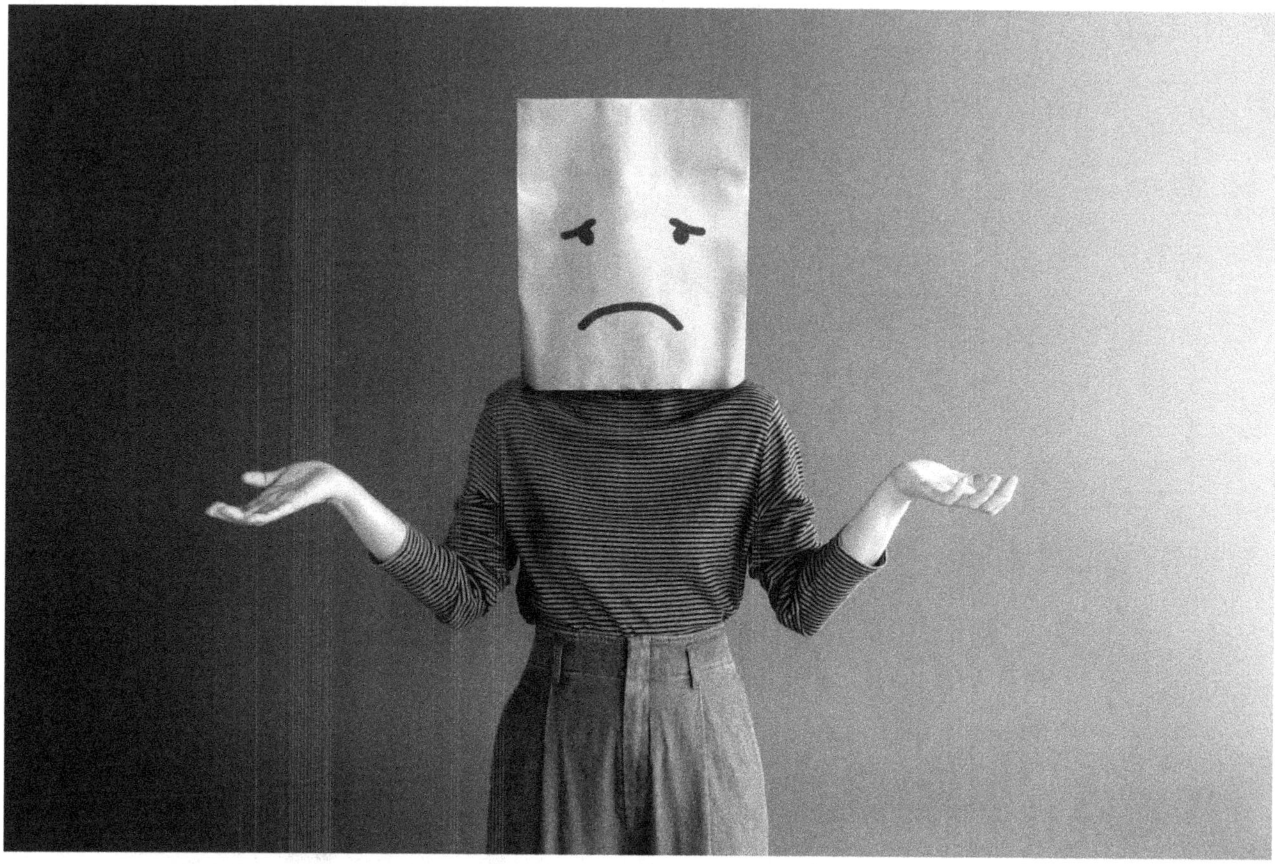

The Anxious Patient

> Many people do not like going to the doctor. (Anecdotally, we know even more dislike visiting their dentist.) Whether they're deeply worried about a condition or fearful of possible treatment, these patients can be classified as anxious.
>
> Anxious patients might be obvious to spot — some will cry or shake, for example. Others display their anxiety in more subtle ways, such as avoiding eye contact or fidgeting. Anxious patients can be too distressed to express their health concerns or to fully absorb important information you give regarding their care.
>
> To effectively care for anxious patients, first **assure them they are in good hands**. Remind them that you specialize in this area of medicine because you want to help individuals just like them. They'll need to feel supported in order to fully comprehend their medical care.
>
> When appropriate, offer sympathy. If you are treating a patient with a chronic condition, for example, you could say: *"I'm sorry you have to go through this. I know it's tough, but it's important to remain hopeful."*
>
> Finally, let them know they can contact you at any time to ask questions or discuss their concerns.[6]

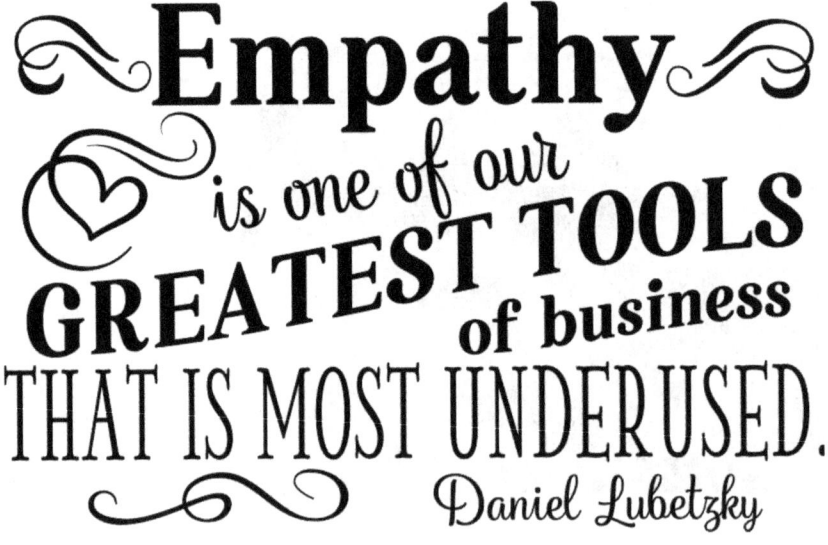

Empathy is one of our GREATEST TOOLS of business THAT IS MOST UNDERUSED.
— Daniel Lubetzky

---

[6] https://www.patientpop.com/blog/running-a-practice/patient-experience/5-strategies-for-dealing-with-problem-patients-and-when-you-should-let-them-go/

Why?

You, as a Chronic Pain employee, likely already know this (I had to learn it by research). I fully understood that depression and chronic pain are so closely connected (I've often joked, "Like 'white' and 'milk', good luck breaking the bond between depression and chronic pain.")

"The association between anxiety disorders and pain may be stronger than the association between depression and pain. (Learn more about the most common anxiety disorders seen in pain patients, as well as new DSM-5 diagnostic criteria.)"[7] (parenthesis added)

Sounds like we can count on anxiety-affected patients as a given in a pain management practice or clinic. According to PSYCOM.net, "Researchers have found that experiencing a chronic illness puts a person at increased risk for developing anxiety or an anxiety disorder. Roughly 40% of people with cancer report experiencing psychological distress that often takes the shape of excessive worry or panic attacks. **People with chronic pain are three times more likely to develop symptoms of anxiety.**"[8] (emphasis added)

How?

How to help a patient struggling with anxiety...

Given the large percentage of pain patients who suffer with anxiety, I imagine you've also attended multi-day conferences dedicated to this subject (in addition to angry patients).

As a specialist in Chronic Pain management, you've likely discovered methods whereby you can assist patients with anxiety to help themselves, locate assistance in the medical community, or to find a support group. You've likely been present when a patient experiences a full-fledged panic attack—perhaps because of a discussion (such as the need to decrease opiates) or before or during a treatment or procedure.

Some people don't like needles.

Others are so distressed by the chronic pain they suffer that the mere thought of additional pain (such as experienced by various therapies or treatments) is more than she can bear.

---

[7] David Cosio, Ph.D., ABPP and Lotus M. Meshreki, Ph.D.; https://www.practicalpainmanagement.com/treatments/psychological/cognitive-behavioral-therapy/anxiety-pain

[8] https://www.psycom.net/chronic-pain-illness-anxiety

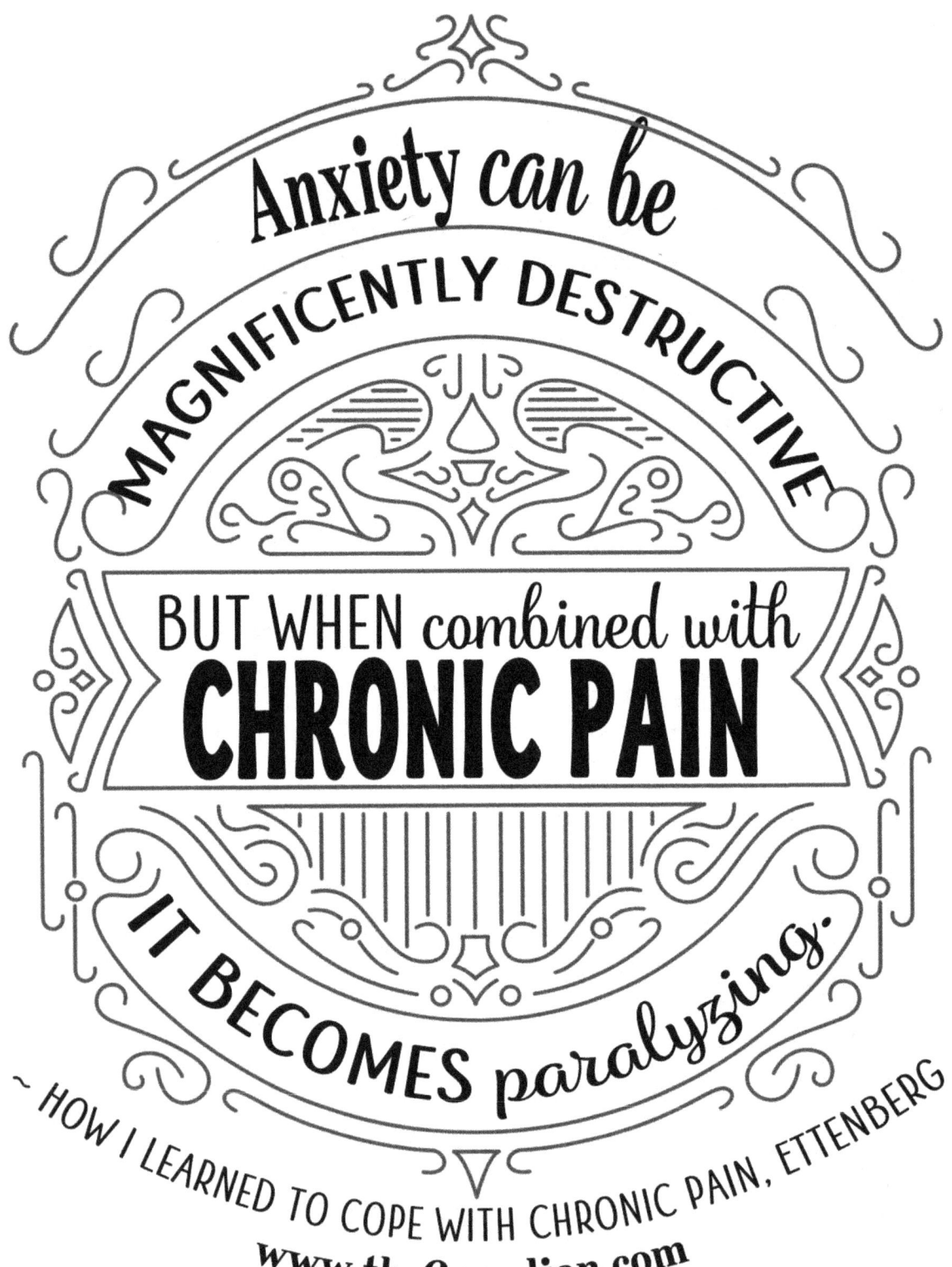

How? continued:
> "Too much anxiety, or anxiety left unchecked, can lead to intense fear that can quickly spin out of control. Anxious thoughts can 'feed' even greater anxious thoughts, or they may stop you so you are unable to function," says pain psychologist Jonas I. Bromberg. "if you have chronic pain, your body and mind may feel under attack. As a result, you are likely to feel worried or apprehensive about many things."[9]

Is it possible to develop a list of Best Practices to empower you to help patients, despite their anxiety?

Best Practices

1. **Listen!** "The most important skill to learn when dealing with anxious patients is to listen. Most people just want to know that you are listening to their concerns."[10]
2. **Empathize!** "Be wary of your own biases or assumptions. Sometimes we have conscious or unconscious beliefs about how people should or should not behave in certain situations. The fact of the matter is that unless you have actually been in this situation yourself, you have no right to judge how someone else should feel or act. Do your best to put yourself in their shoes."[11]
3. **Compliment the doctor's (or NP's) strengths** to the patient; express confidence in him/her.
4. **Refrain from expressing doubts** or concerns or lack of confidence in a provider.
5. **Recognize that a percentage of all patients suffer anxiety associated with doctors' offices**. Sometimes this is a result of past experiences (painful or otherwise unpleasant) in doctors' offices, and sometimes upon assumptions about a scheduled treatment. The fear of the needle might prove a greater hurdle than the pain caused by the actual needle.
6. **Validate feelings.** Patients are allowed to feel whatever it is they feel. Telling someone "don't be afraid" won't change the fact that they are, indeed, afraid. All the statement does is tell the patient "you're not allowed to be the way you are"—a hot spot in today's world (and a sure-fire way to wave a large flag announcing you don't comprehend the patient's circumstances).
    a. Validation *does not equal* agreement. You're simply acknowledging the words or emotions of the client.
    b. "I see you're anxious."

---

[9] http://princessinthetower.org/when-chronic-pain-increases-anxiety-with-tools-to-calm-soothe/

[10] https://www.travelnursing.org/7-ways-to-provide-exceptional-patient-care/

[11] https://www.travelnursing.org/7-ways-to-provide-exceptional-patient-care/

7. **Do Not Say: "Calm down."** A person in the throes of an anxiety attack is adrift on a tide of adrenalin and cortisol (the stress hormones).
8. **"Rather than minimize their experience** ("There's nothing to be afraid of."), **focus on normalizing anxiety and using supportive phrases** ("Many of my patients have concerns similar to yours.") **Normalizing** anxiety **shows empathy** and helps the patient understand that they are not alone in experiencing anxiety."[12]
9. "Reduce anxiety by **introducing yourself and your role** and orienting patients and families to whatever is to follow. Focus on patients by asking questions about their work, children and aspects of their personal lives, which may also help keep patients calm. the message, here, too, is that **you are interested in them as people, not just as patients**. (Crystal Gustafson (2015))."[13] (emphasis added)
10. **Patients want to be believed.** When in their own minds, through their own emotional lens, they wholly believe *they're telling the simple* truth about their pain and circumstances to their healthcare provider, they are desperate to have their pain concerns legitimized.
    a. What if you, as any member of the healthcare team in Chronic Pain doubt that the patient's condition is as bad as she says? Is there a best practice in that circumstance? _____

    b. If you can't say "I believe you," what can you say?
    _____

---

[12] https://aestheticsjournal.com/feature/managing-anxious-patients

[13] https://www.nurse.com/blog/2016/11/11/how-nurses-can-help-reduce-their-patients-anxiety/

Excellent Resources

Scan QR code OR type the following link into your search window:

Depression and Anxiety in Pain, PMC, US National Library of Medicine National Institutes of Health
https://www.ncbi.nlm.nih.gov/pmc/articles/PMC4590059/

Scan QR code OR type the following link into your search window:

http://www.instituteforchronicpain.org/understanding-chronic-pain/complications/anxiety

Treating co-occurring chronic low back pain & generalized anxiety disorder, 2.0 CE hours, 0.5 Rx Contact Hours.

Scan QR code OR type the following link into your search window:

https://nursing.ceconnection.com/ovidfiles/00006205-201601000-00003.pdf

As the url (address) for this resource is so long (and too gnarly to type), I recommend "Googling" the phrase "Universal Upset Patient Protocol" OR scanning the QR code.

> "Your Smile is your logo, your PERSONALITY is your business card, how you leave others feeling after having an expereince with you becomes your trademark."
>
> ANONYMOUS

Chapter Seven
7/10 mile: Need a Break? Step Away. Breathe.

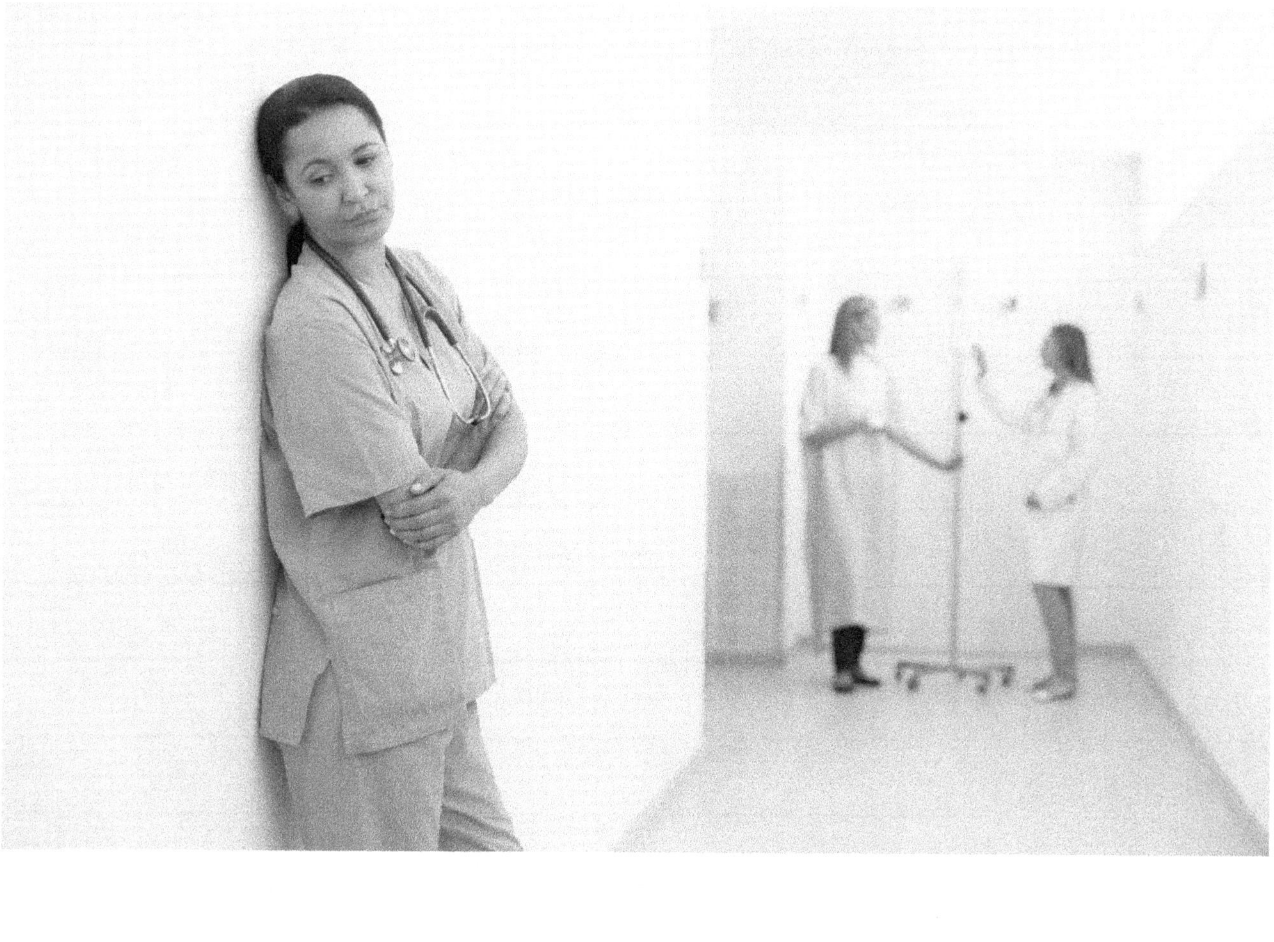

Compassion Fatigue

Compassion Fatigue in your specialty—chronic pain—is very real.

With respectful acknowledgment, we'll note that Compassion Fatigue is not this training's main focus.

"In fact, I believe today's message can *help*. It surely can't hurt." ~ Kristin Holt, RN

Thoughts:

_____
_____
_____
_____
_____
_____
_____
_____
_____
_____
_____
_____

Chapter Eight
8/10 mile: Three Simple Tools

If three simple tools could *reduce your burdens*, elevate your mood, increase job satifaction, and reduce the "chafe" of these challenges...

...would you use them?

The three tools I'm about to share with you are tools I've put to use since L&D and patients in pain, and I put them to use to ensure every WW meeting I lead and every person I met *had the best I had to offer.*

I cared about my people.

The most beautiful, synergistic thing happened. Not only did my people benefit the way I wanted and needed them to... but I found my personal rewards were enormous. And just for me.

Here, I thought I'd been generous, gracious, giving... and my own job satisfaction soared. Like a smile, you can't really give a positive attitude away. Smiles and positive attitudes linger and strengthen and benefit the giver.

There's my self-endorsement. Call me a "celebrity endorsement" if that helps you want to jump on the bandwagon.

Do it for yourself if you won't do it for your coworkers and especially if you won't do it for your patients.

No matter what you do after this hour together is through, I urge you to commit to trying these three Tools (or Strategies) on for size, and at least, experimenting to see if they work.

I challenge you to observe with care and look for ways to adopt these simple tools. Within reason, make them your own.

I'm confident each of these simple strategies will reduce your angst with the job. You'll go home at night with a smile on your face—and a joyful glow about your heart. And that warm, amazing realization that **you've made a difference in the lives of real people**—people whose circumstances could've easily been your own. You realize that, don't you? That whatever elements of fate or statistics or whatever pulled my name out of the hat as a long-time chronic pain sufferer just as easily could've picked YOU.

What if?

What if you were the one in pain, and not me?

What if you were the patient at the pain clinic where you now work?

What if you had close-up familiarity with what pain does to a person?

What if chronic pain had stolen one too many things from you to date, and you'd simply HAD IT. You're hanging by a thread, desperate, with emotions so near the surface, you fear you'll embarrass yourself with tears of frustration.

I already know the answer to "what if".

You'd want the best. You'd want someone to answer your questions, to anticipate questions you hadn't thought to ask—or those you were too scared to ask—and ensure you're well cared for.

You'd want someone to show compassion and understanding with your limitations.

You'd want a soft voice and words of encouragement.

You'd want to be treated with courtesy and respect. You'd want your provider to listen and ask questions until you're both understanding each other.

You'd CRAVE precisely what these three simple tools (call them strategies if you wish) will do for you as the patient.

I promise you'll love what these three simple strategies will do you for you as the Pain Management employee.

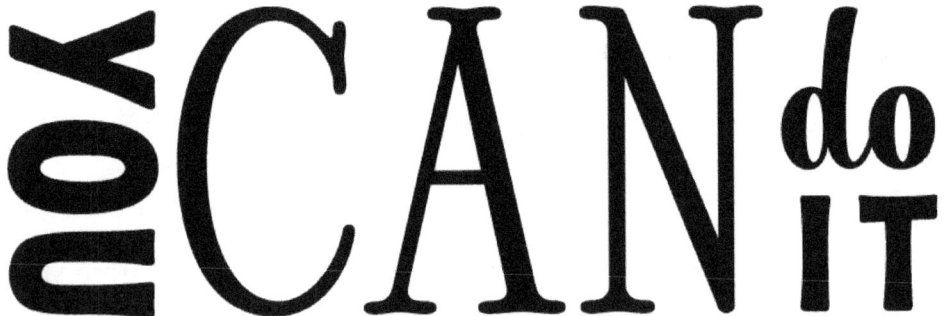

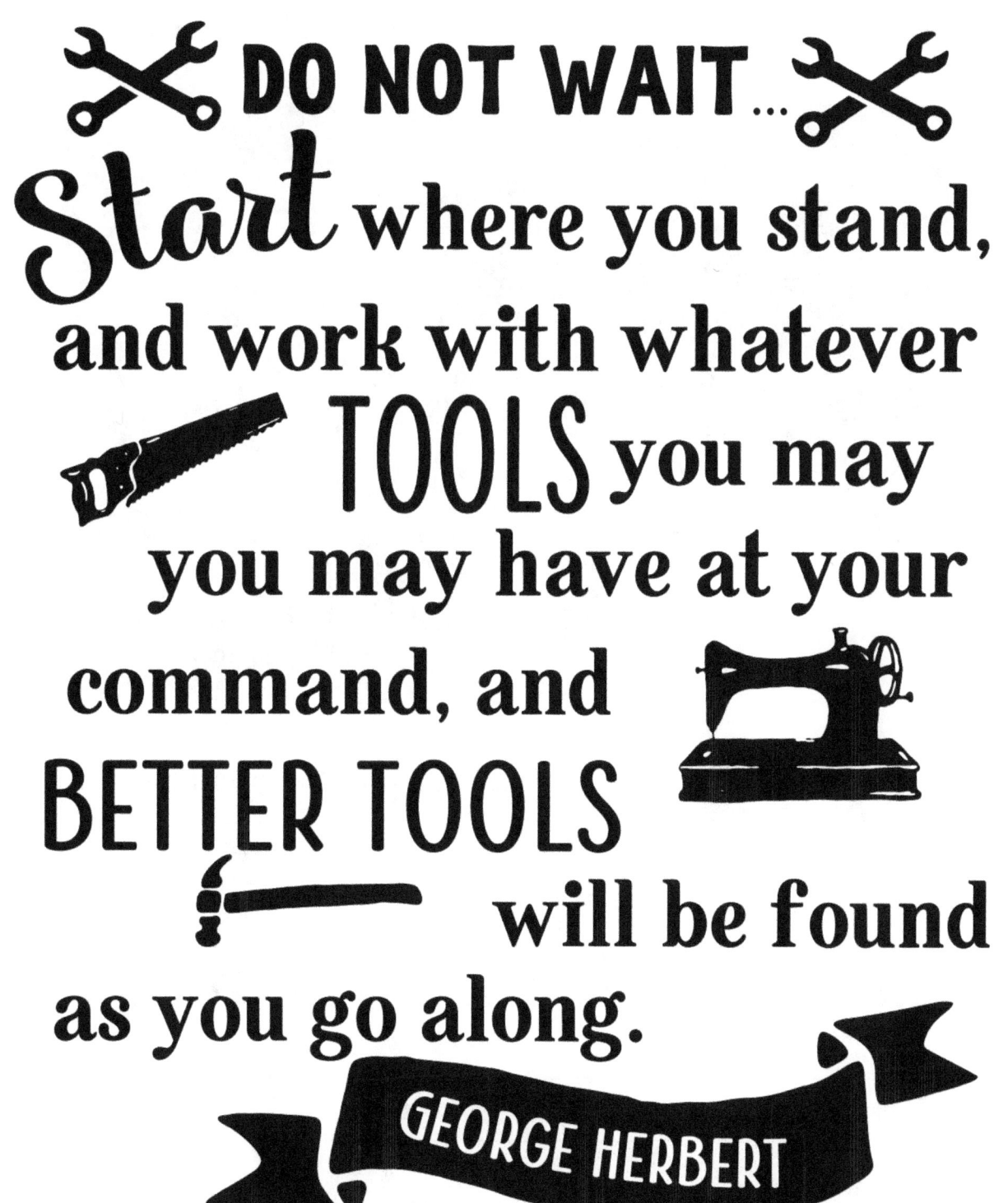

Tool (Strategy) #1: Leave Your Stuff At The Door

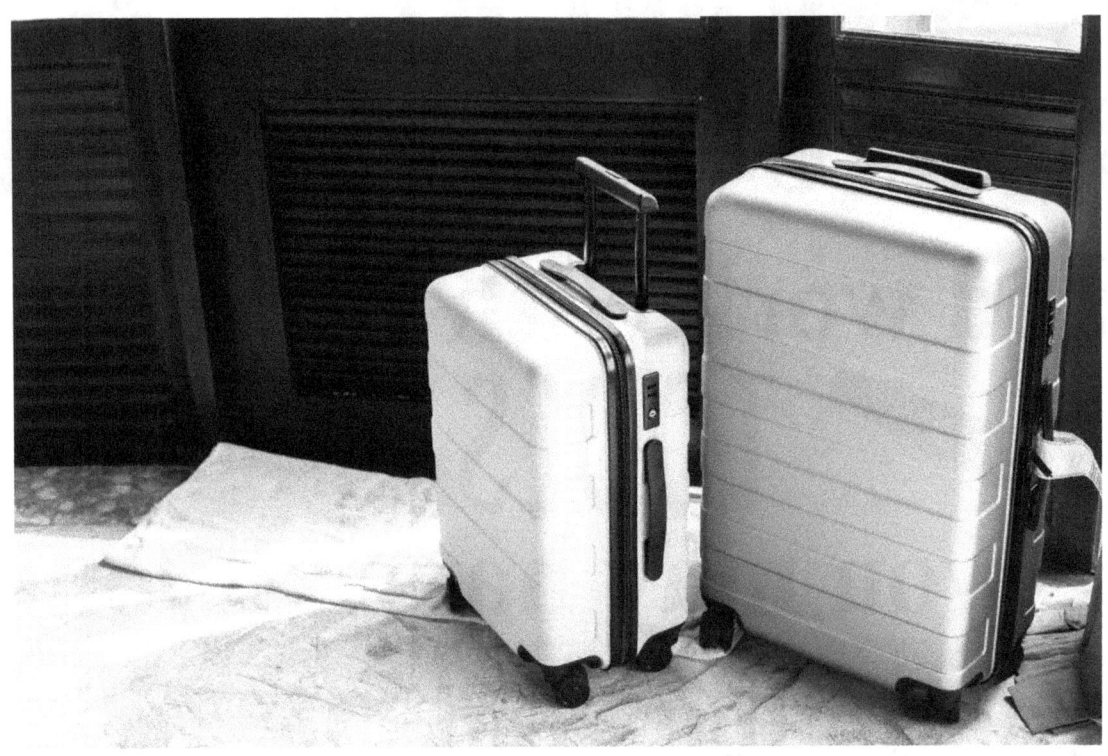

Professionalism = leaving your stuff at the door, as this frees you up to be FULLY PRESENT.

If you must, Fake It 'til you Make It.

Am I good at leaving my stuff at the door? An example:

_____

_____

_____

_____

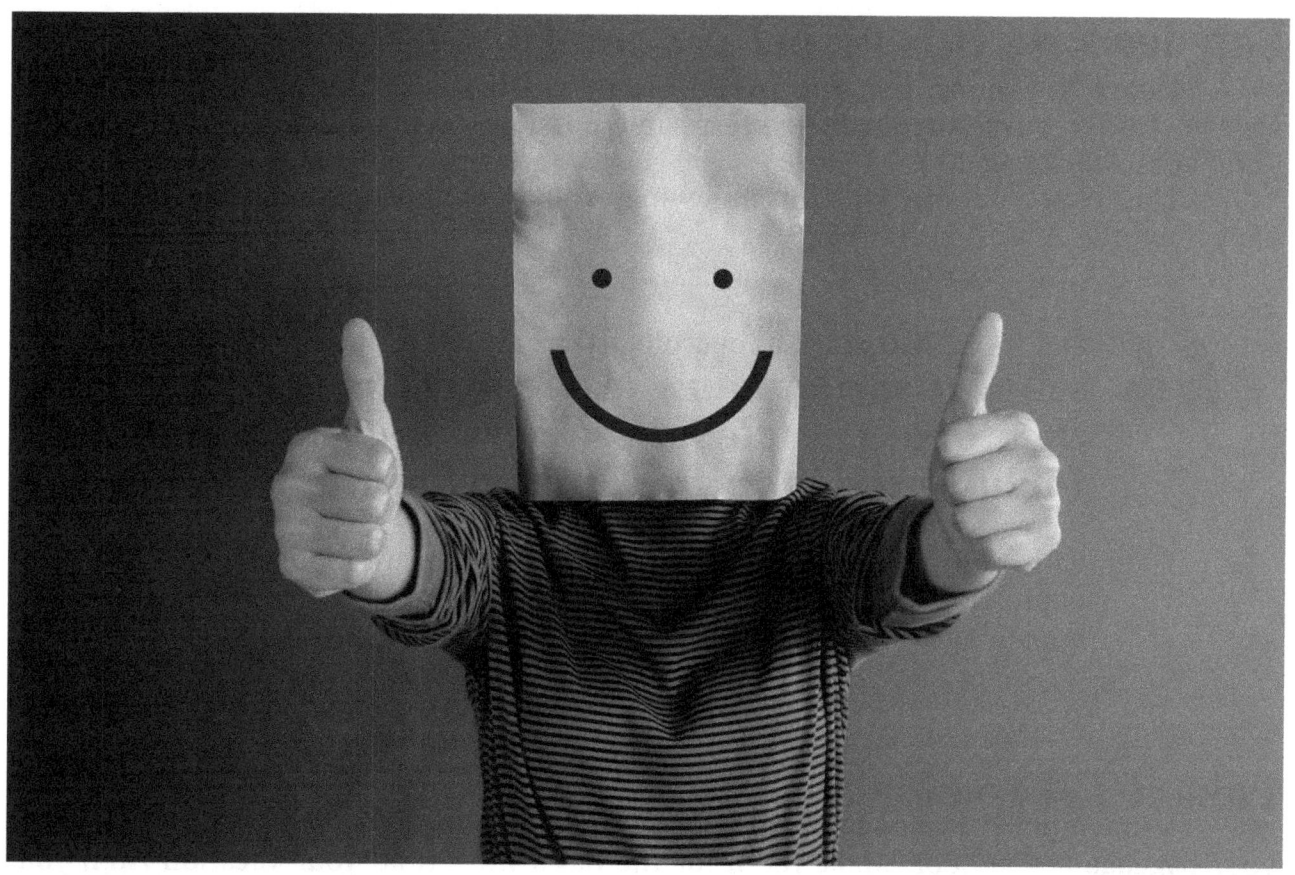

What's In it For Me?

No matter how you're feeling when you get to work– **LEAVE YOUR NEGATIVE FEELINGS AT THE DOOR.**

I know, you're asking: I see how this helps the PATIENTS, but how is this a payoff for me?

Consider this analogy:

If you don't Leave Your Stuff At The Door, you're tromping inside, continuing to wear your farmer's boots straight from the cow pen and milking shed into the front parlor. Without so much as using the boot scraper.

Come on, cowboy! Take off those filthy boots at the door, and come on in. Put on the clean boots waiting for you here. Likewise, **don't carry the dirt of the workday into your home and to impact the ones you love**. Learning to separate the two will bless your life in myriad ways.

Science says this effort is good for you

"Science has shown that **the mere act of smiling** can **lift your mood, lower stress, boost your immune system** and possibly even **prolong your life**."[14] ~ (emphasis added)

What? Wait a minute. Isn't this all wrong? You thought people smile *because* they're happy, not the other way around.

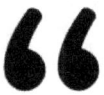 **Dr. Isha Gupta**[15] a neurologist from IGEA Brain and Spine explains ***a smile spurs a chemical reaction in the brain, releasing certain hormones including dopamine and serotonin.*** "Dopamine increases our feelings of happiness. Serotonin release is associated with reduced stress. Low levels of serotonin are associated with depression and aggression," says Dr. Gupta. "Low levels of dopamine are also associated with depression."[16] (emphasis added)

Fake It Till You Make It

If you're not in the mood to smile when you arrive at work—remember to check all of your baggage at the door. Make room for the day's work (and your vacation from your own troubles) by making yourself fully present.

Let your body's mood-regulating hormones benefit, measurably, by your choice to smile, to say hello, to greet patients with professional courtesy and kindness.

Feeling grumpy? Let your serotonin rise!

Wishing you were somewhere else? Pretend there's nowhere else you'd rather be. Show your coworkers and your patients that you're committed to being fully present and determined to help.

---

[14] https://www.nbcnews.com/better/health/smiling-can-trick-your-brain-happiness-boost-your-health-ncna822591

[15] https://www.igeaneuro.com/specialties/neurology/

[16] https://www.nbcnews.com/better/health/smiling-can-trick-your-brain-happiness-boost-your-health-ncna822591

Excellent Resources

Scan QR code OR type the following link into your search window:

https://www.inc.com/kevin-daum/5-ways-to-leave-your-personal-stress-at-home-where-it-belongs.html

Scan QR code OR type the following link into your search window:

https://www.forbes.com/sites/rachelritlop/2016/11/15/how-millennials-can-stop-personal-issues-from-affecting-their-work/#1f2836392ea9

Scan QR code OR type the following link into your search window:

https://workplace.stackexchange.com/questions/34846/how-to-leave-home-personal-life-issues-at-home-and-focus-on-work-while-at-work

Scan QR code OR type the following link into your search window:

https://hbr.org/2016/07/dont-take-work-stress-home-with-you

Scan QR code OR type the following link into your search window:

https://www.quora.com/How-do-you-keep-your-personal-problems-from-affecting-your-work-performance

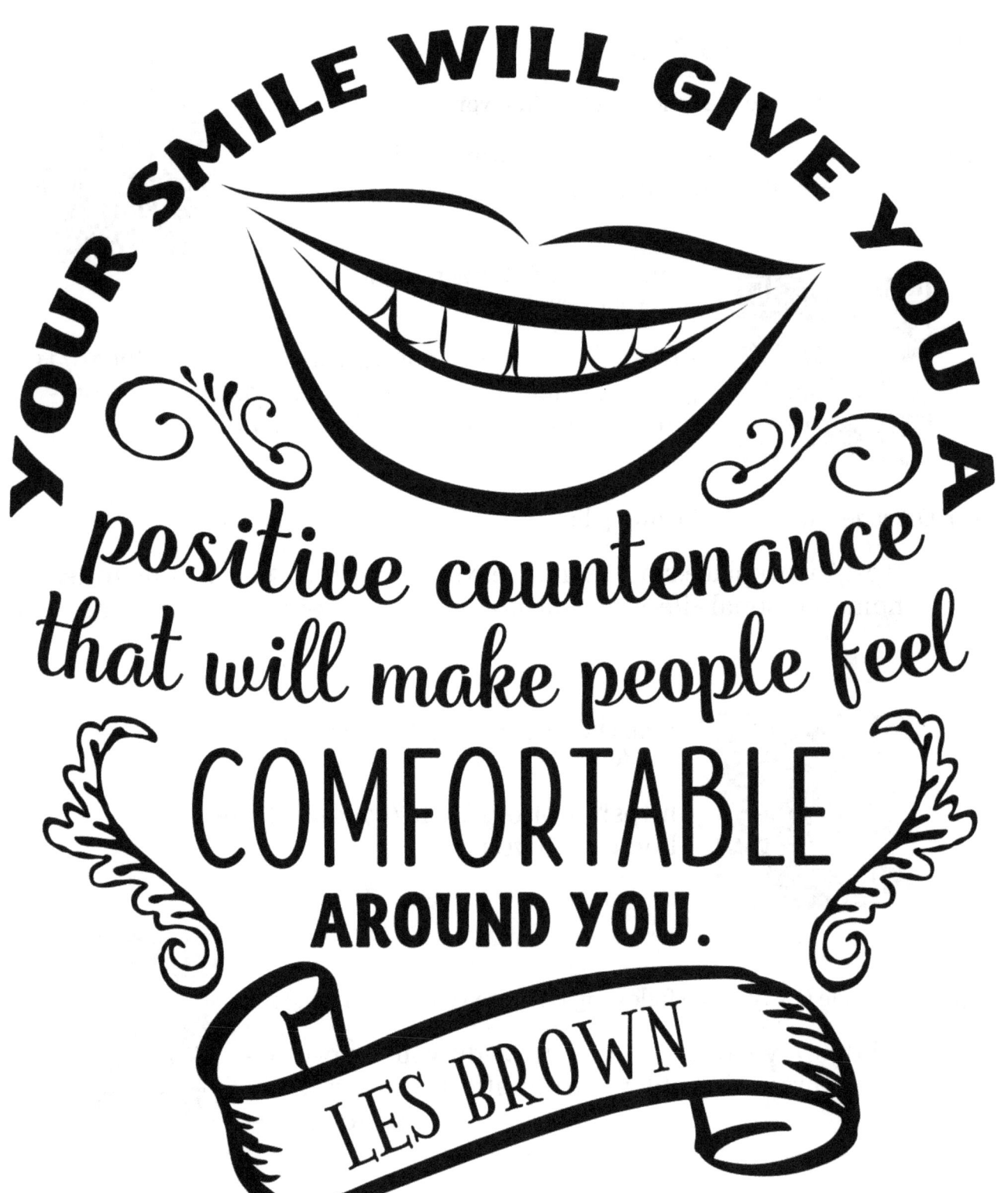

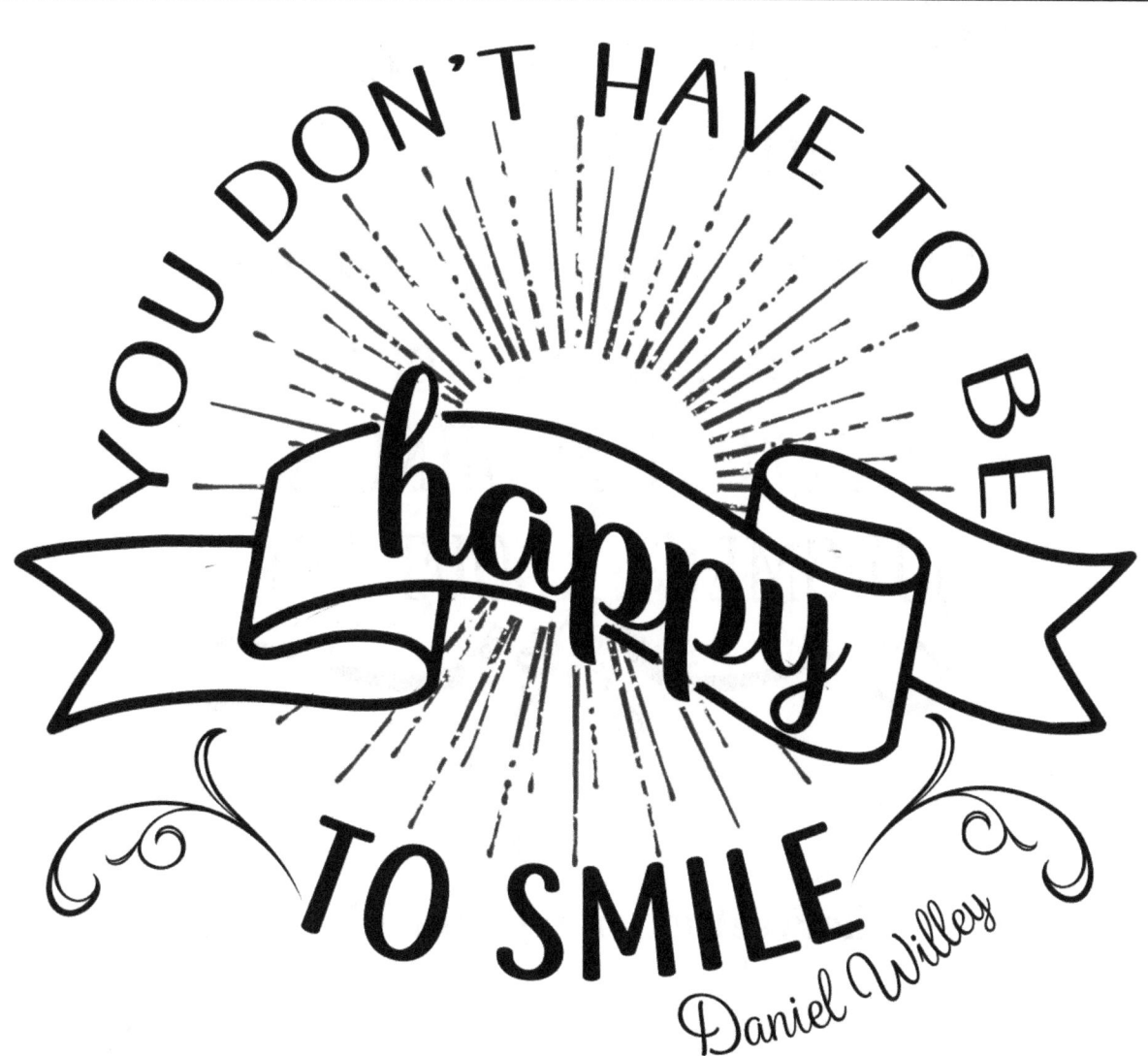

"You don't have to be happy to smile"
— Daniel Willey

To walk a mile in (someone's) shoes:

To spend time TRYING TO CONSIDER or UNDERSTAND ANOTHER PERSON'S perspectives, experiences, or motivations BEFORE MAKING A JUDGMENT ABOUT THEM.

TheFreeDictionary.com, Idioms

Tool (Strategy) #2: Empathy/Sympathy/Compassion

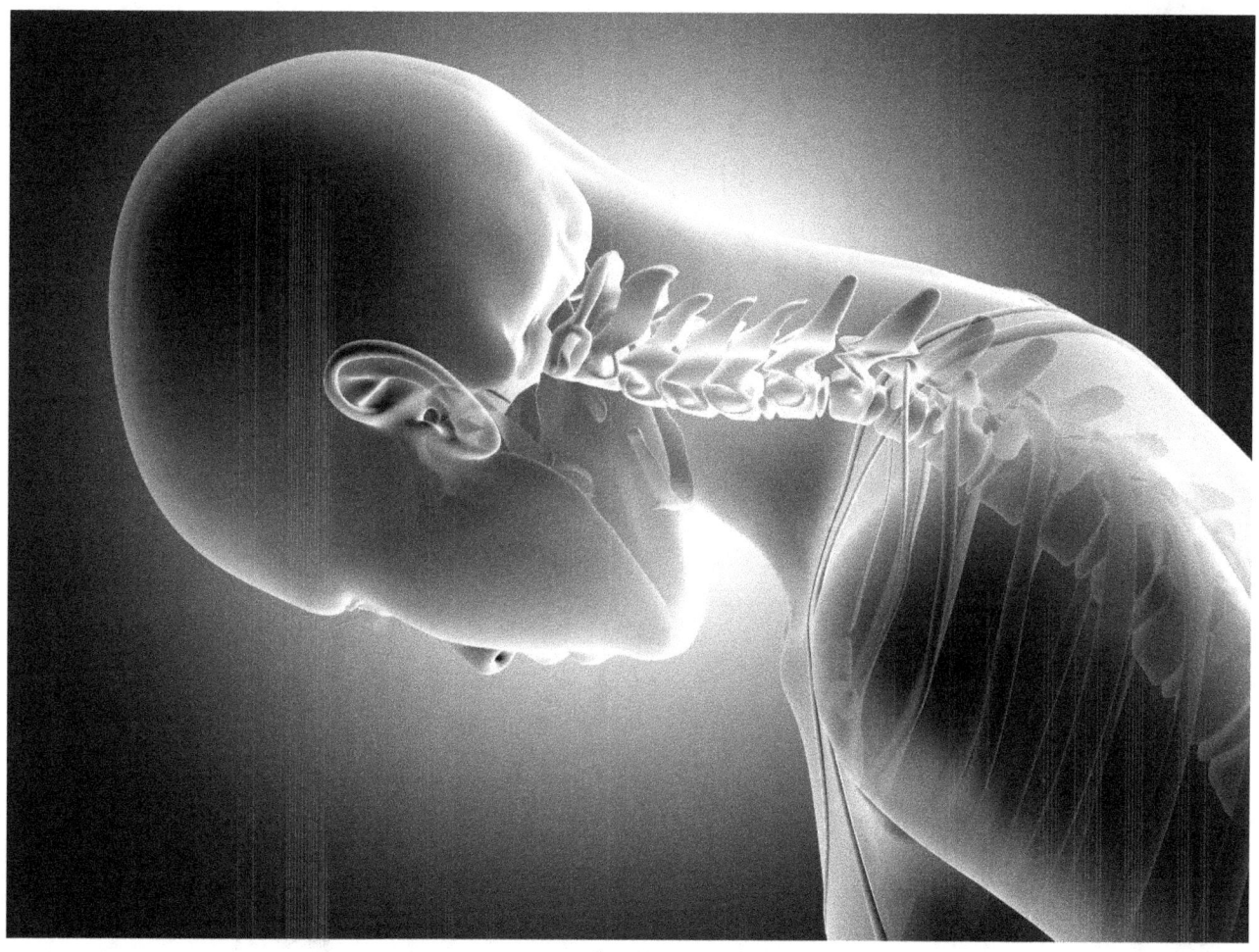

Definitions aside, the key is to pause, consider, reflect, and see the world through your patient's eyes.

> Could a greater miracle take place than for us to look through each other's eyes for an instant.
>
> — Henry David Thoreau

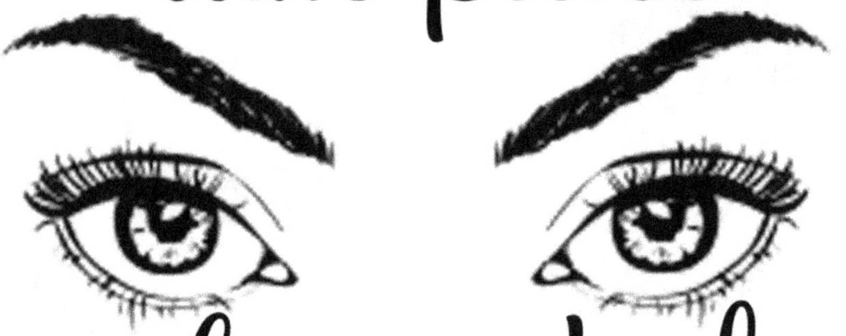

Video Clip: What is the Patient's Name?

(scan the QR code to view the video on YouTube, or transcribe the link—beware the link *is case sensitive*)

https://www.youtube.com/watch?v=zfpT_ppKuos

Thoughts:

_____
_____
_____
_____
_____
_____
_____
_____
_____
_____

Listening is the art of ENTERING THE SKIN OF THE OTHER AND WEARING IT for a time as if it were YOUR OWN.

— David Spangler

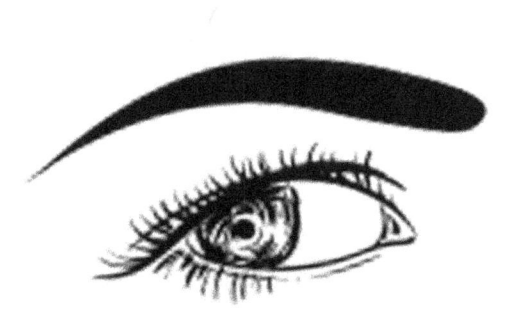
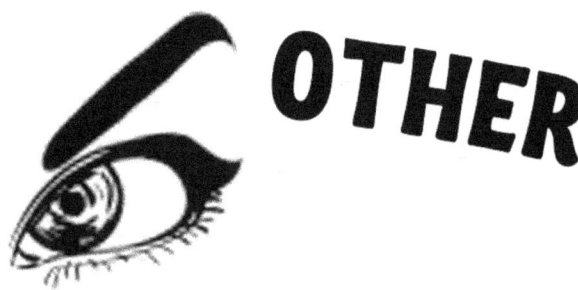

People Who Read...

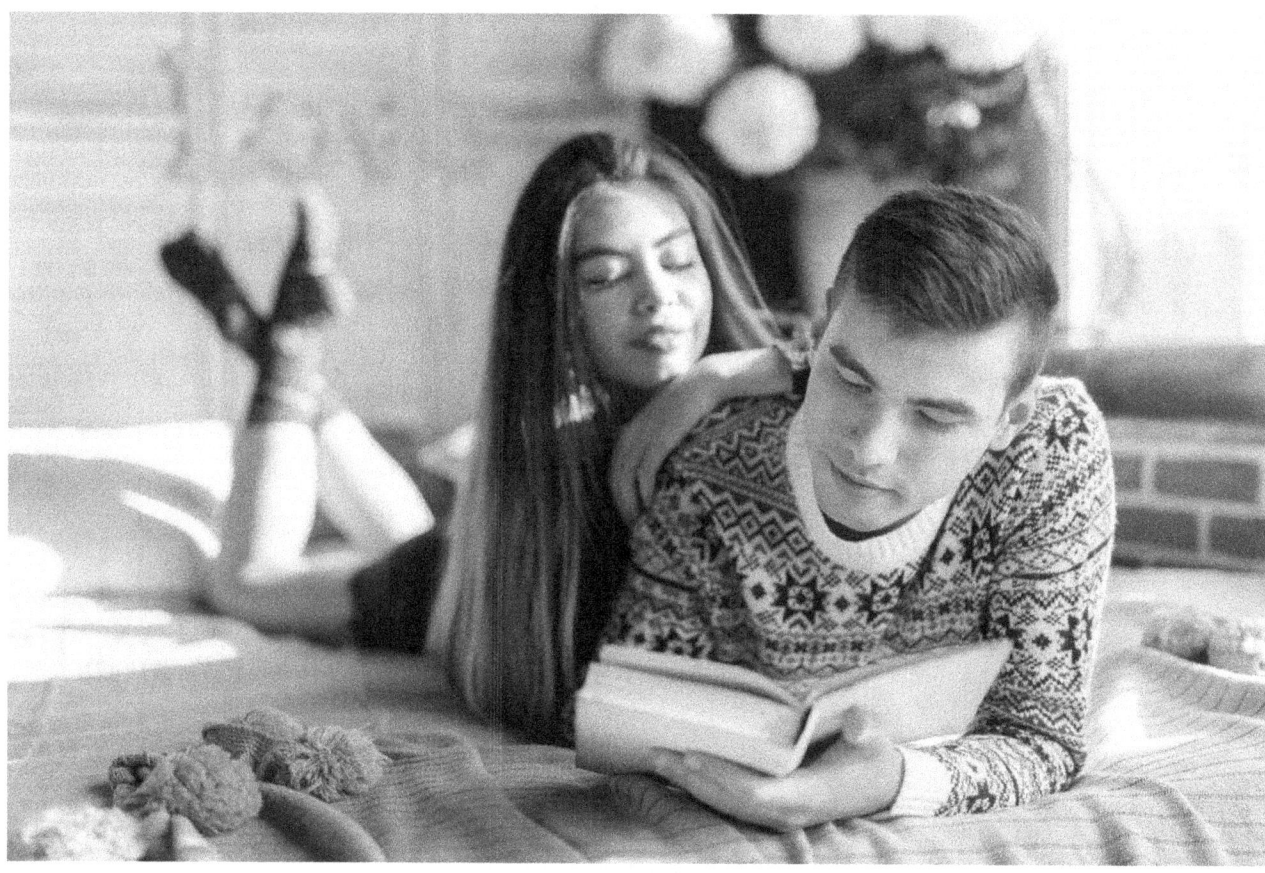

According to *Scientific American*[17]
Readers of FICTION make far better husbands, boyfriends, wives, girlfriends...
Because readers, by chance of their glimpses of alternate points of view and myriad motivations for behavior, are more able to have compassion for others.

Do *you* read fiction? More than one book a month? How about nonfiction titles? If you read at least one book per month, good for you! "Readers" are among the most imaginative, who most easily understand someone else's unique and differing viewpoint.

---

[17] https://www.scientificamerican.com/article/novel-finding-reading-literary-fiction-improves-empathy/

You CAN empathize with patients' experiences, good *and* bad.

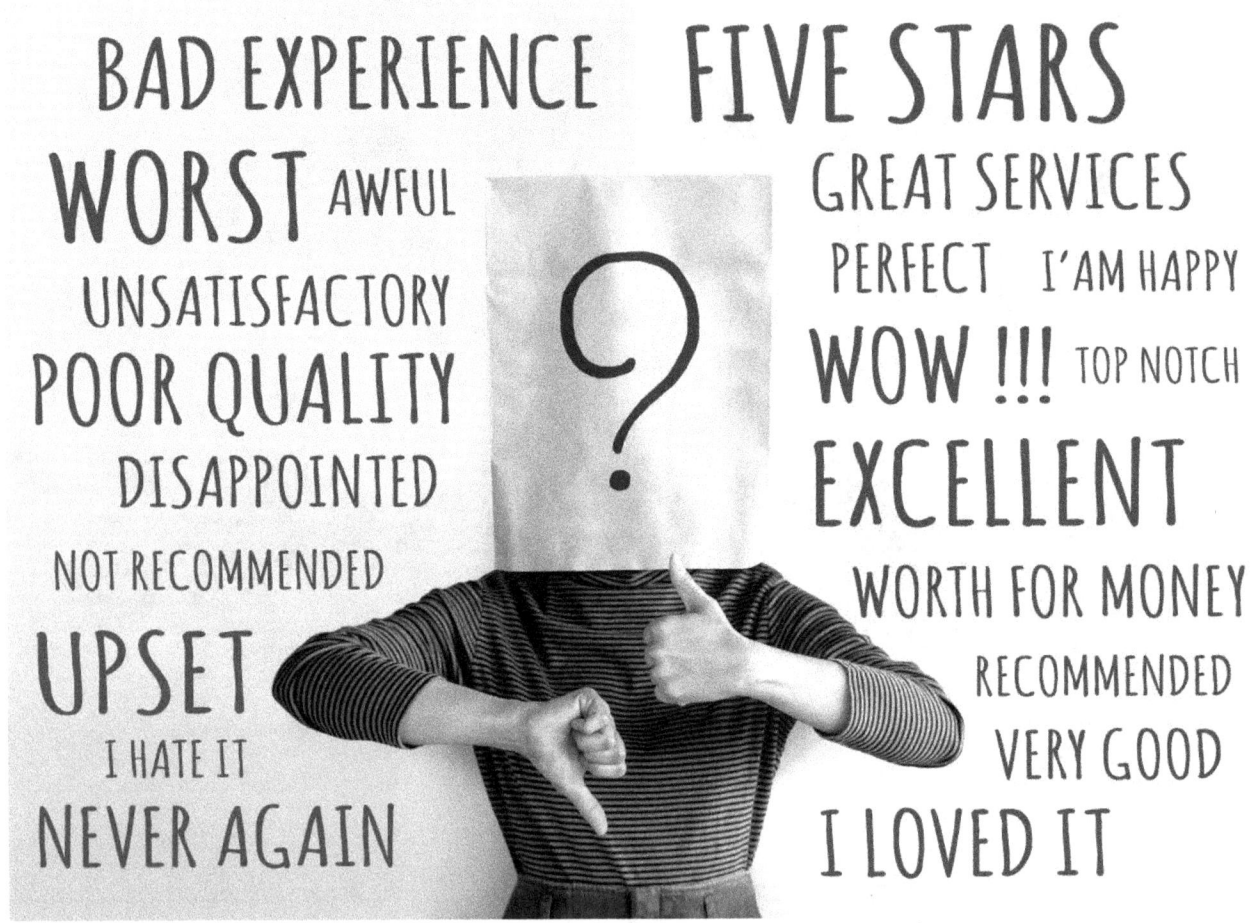

You have had your own WORST EVER and BEST EVER experiences with customer service, no matter which side of the equation you were on (employee or client).

It's All About How You Make Them Feel

It's not about whether you could bend or break the rules…
It's not about the refund or lack thereof…
It's not about the clinic and the providers running behind schedule.
It's not about the plan to reduce opioid medications.
Ultimately, it's all about how you made them feel.
Did she feel heard? Acknowledged? Understood?
Did he feel like an individual? Or like he was a mere number?

> PEOPLE WILL FORGET what you said. THEY WILL FORGET what you did. BUT THEY WILL NEVER FORGET how you made them FEEL.
>
> *Maya Angelou*

Video Clip: The Human Connection to Patient Care

(scan the QR code to view the video on YouTube, or transcribe the link—beware the link *is case sensitive*)

https://www.youtube.com/watch?v=cDDWvj_q-o8&t=4s&index=5&list=PLbiVpU59JkVb_ROoQuQnIlAHAeFUKgUhf

Thoughts:

___
___
___
___
___
___
___
___
___

Tool (Strategy) #3: Kindness

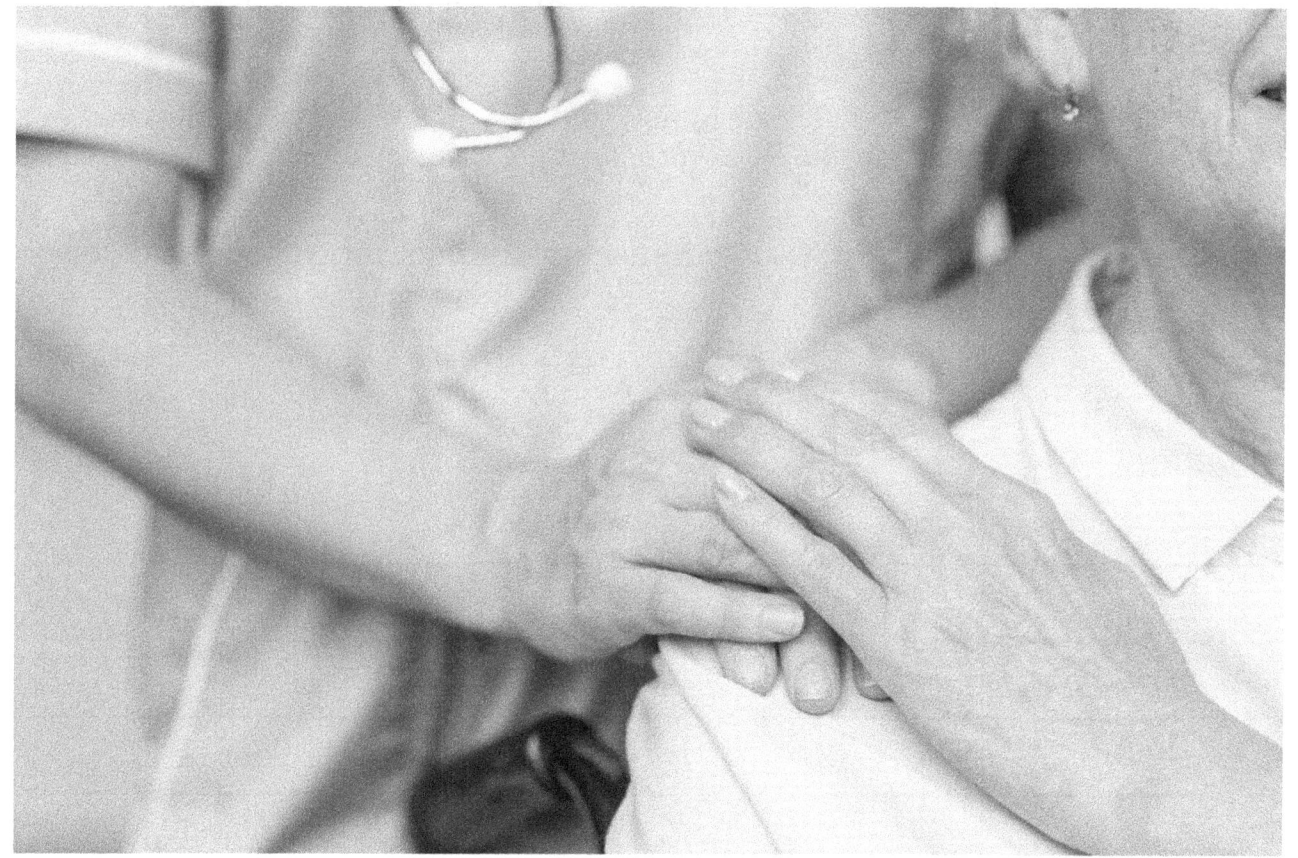

BE KIND *for everyone you meet is fighting a hard battle.*
— IAN MACLAREN

What's In it For Me?
Did you know? Science proved exercising kindness pays off.

 (scan the QR code to view the video on Random Acts of Kindness, or transcribe the link—*this one is not* case sensitive)

https://www.randomactsofkindness.org/the-science-of-kindness

Thoughts:

_____
_____
_____
_____
_____
_____
_____
_____
_____

KINDNESS
as simple as...

1. Fully Present
2. Genuine, Active Listening
3. Validation
4. What Can I Say?
5. Quality Customer Care
6.
7.
8.
9.
10.
11.
12.

Kindness

1. **Fully Present**
   1. No personal conversations in front of patients.
   2. Body language cues
   3. Look up. "Thank you for your patience. We'll be with you as quickly as possible."
   4. Give the client/patient you're with your full attention.
   5. Reflect their general mood and energy level.
      1. To be bubbly sunshine when the patient is somber and frightened carries a sense of cluelessness (or lack of understanding).
      2. Don't assume a set of circumstances (or a situation the patient is in the process of relaying to you) is good or bad until the client tells you her judgment. A judgment based on your personal POV is a great way to show the client you're dissimilar, not listening, or of different beliefs.
2. **Genuine, Active Listening**
   1. Eye contact
   2. Responses ("Say more", "I'm listening, "Yes?")
   3. LISTEN *far* more than you SPEAK.
   4. YOUR body language– look at them, turn your whole body or head toward them when they speak. You may want to stop what you're otherwise doing. If that's not possible, make sure you look periodically at the person you're listening to and use other cues to show you're paying attention.
   5. Answer questions when asked, and...
   6. Ask clarifying questions (AND AVOID INTERRUPTING!—unless this has all gone on far too long), especially "Say More" and questions that clarify the moral good/bad judgment the CLIENT has made, and to verify that what YOU think you heard is indeed what the patient meant to convey.
   7. Rather than formulating your reply as the client is speaking, L I S T E N....
   8. Do they need <u>acknowledgment</u> or <u>validation</u>?
   9. Reflect back to them their words and feelings, "I'm hearing you say... Am I understanding?" Or something super brief when the client pauses: "You were afraid." You're likely to hear verbal agreement, which makes the client feel like you were really listening.
3. **Validation**
   1. LISTEN WITHOUT INTERRUPTION. (120 seconds may be ALL the patient needs; you can afford 120 seconds to fully understand the problem, to meet the patient halfway, and to ensure that his needs are met accurately and well– in one brief and simple act of kindness.
   2. Do not make "Silver Lining Comments" ("I miscarried." "At least you know you can have children."; "Bob and I are having marriage trouble." "At least you have a marriage.")

3. <u>You're not necessarily agreeing</u>– you're simply validating the person's feelings and statements. You're acknowledging you've heard.
4. **Validation** is the recognition and acceptance of another person's thoughts, feelings, sensations, and behaviors as understandable. (Psychology today)
    1. Works best when fully present. Give all of your attention, from eye contact to active listening skills, to that person.
    2. Validation can be non-verbal. A nod, a thumbs-up, a smile, etc.
    3. Validation can be verbal (and sometimes it needs to be). "Yes." "Congratulations! I knew you could do it." "
5. Accurate **Reflection**. Infuse this reflection of what you've heard with authenticity. If your expectation is to truly understand without judgment, the client will feel validated.
6. **Mindreading**: Guess at the other person's feelings or thoughts, based upon what they've said and their body language. Some people can't acknowledge their feelings or emotions, and may be unclear about what it is they're feeling or thinking... and "mindreading" reflects back a reasonable assumption for assessment. The person might disagree with you, but at least he's now thinking about it.
7. **Self-disclosures, where appropriate**– as a connection in like experiences build connections, trust, and willingness to follow.

4. **What can I say?**
    1. Sometimes, "There are no words."
    2. "I'm sorry."
    3. "I'm so glad you told me. Thank you for trusting me with this."
    4. "I'm here."
    5. "I see how <u>frustrated</u> you are." (angry, upset, fearful, happy --fill in the blank)

5. **Quality Customer Care**
    1. Golden Rule – Absolutely, yes. "Do unto others as you would have others do to you." Imagine for a moment what it would be like for YOU and ME to trade places, Freaky Friday style. Now I'm the pain management clinic's employee and you are the patient.
        1. You enter through the main doors into the lobby and see me behind the reception desk. What would you like to have happen?
        2. You kept your appointment today at the pain clinic. Wearing scrubs, I go through our routine monthly questions with you. What do you want our interaction to look like?
    2. No matter how grumpy, stoic, quiet, nervous, fearful the patients are– ***you have the chance to MAKE A DIFFERENCE.***
        1. Smile.
        2. Inform.
        3. Say good morning or good afternoon.
        4. If you're not able to assist someone right away– tell them so!

5. If you're the ONE interaction a suffering person experiences today, make it the *best* possible.

ALWAYS find OPPORTUNITIES TO MAKE SOMEONE SMILE AND TO OFFER random Acts of kindness IN EVERYDAY life.

~ ROY T. BENNETT

> *Body language and tone of voice — NOT WORDS — are our most POWERFUL ASSESSMENT Tools.*
> — Christopher Voss

Video Clip: Be Kind. Always. Even when serving school lunch.

(scan the QR code to view the video on YouTube, or transcribe the link—take care, as this link *is* case sensitive)

https://www.youtube.com/watch?v=3NGmvynEmwc&index=4&list=PLbiVpU59JkVb_ROoQuQnIlAHAeFUKgUhf
(note: timestamp 4:00 to 6:00 only)

Thoughts:

_____
_____
_____
_____
_____
_____
_____
_____
_____
_____
_____
_____

**Is there a time when at work MY words, actions, response, or body language were unkind? What were the circumstances? How did I feel?
[What did a lack of KINDNESS do <u>to</u> me?]**

_____
_____
_____
_____
_____
_____
_____
_____
_____
_____
_____
_____
_____
_____
_____

Is there a time when MY kindness and shining customer care made ME feel great? What were the circumstances? How did I feel? [What did KINDNESS do _for me_?]

Chapter Nine
9/10 mile: Commitment to Try the Tools

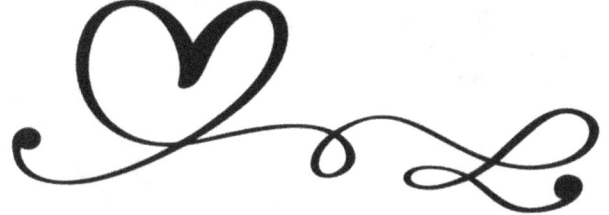

I HEREBY PROMISE THAT I WILL TRY EACH TOOL INDIVIDUALLY AND IN COMBINATION WITH EACH OTHER. I WILL REMIND MYSELF WHAT'S IN IT FOR ME!

_____

my signature

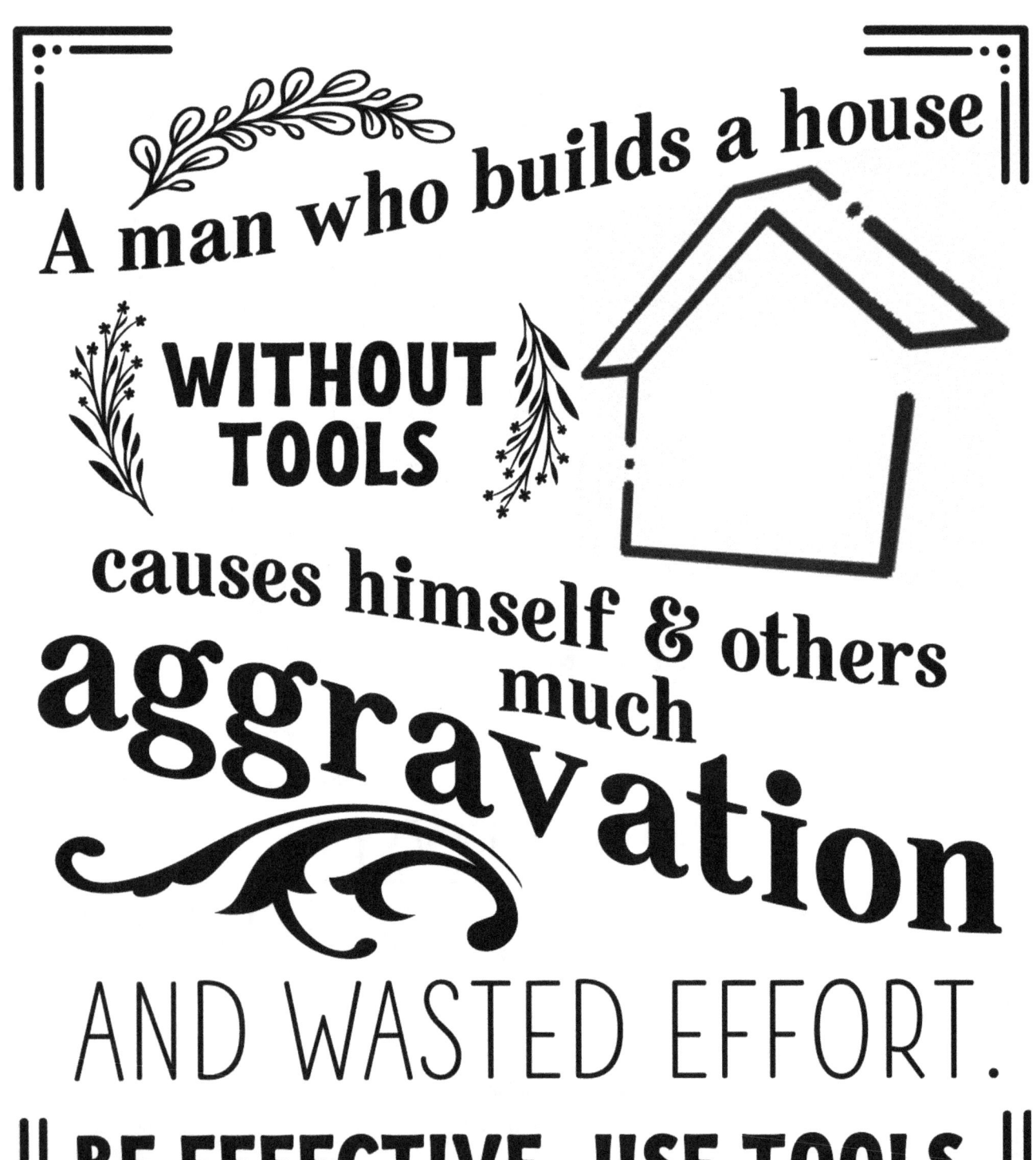

Chapter Ten
10/10 mile: Important Questions

How would I feel if I were the one waiting?
_____
_____
_____
_____

How would I react if I were the one in pain?
_____
_____
_____

Do I take great care with my appearance when I feel crummy?
_____
_____
_____

Am I comfortable showing compassion for those in pain?

_____
_____
_____

Does my impatience show?

_____
_____
_____

Do I have a "smile" in my voice? Explain!

_____
_____
_____

Do I smile at patients? Often, sometimes, never--and why?

_____
_____
_____
_____

Are my listening skills up to par? _____

_____

_____

Do my actions convey compassion? Why or why not?

_____

_____

_____

If it were my mother or sister or best friend or child here for an appointment, would my interaction with the client be different? How so? Why?

_____

_____

_____

ONE thing I want to do differently~ _____

_____

_____

What does KINDNESS look like in this clinic?

Thank You

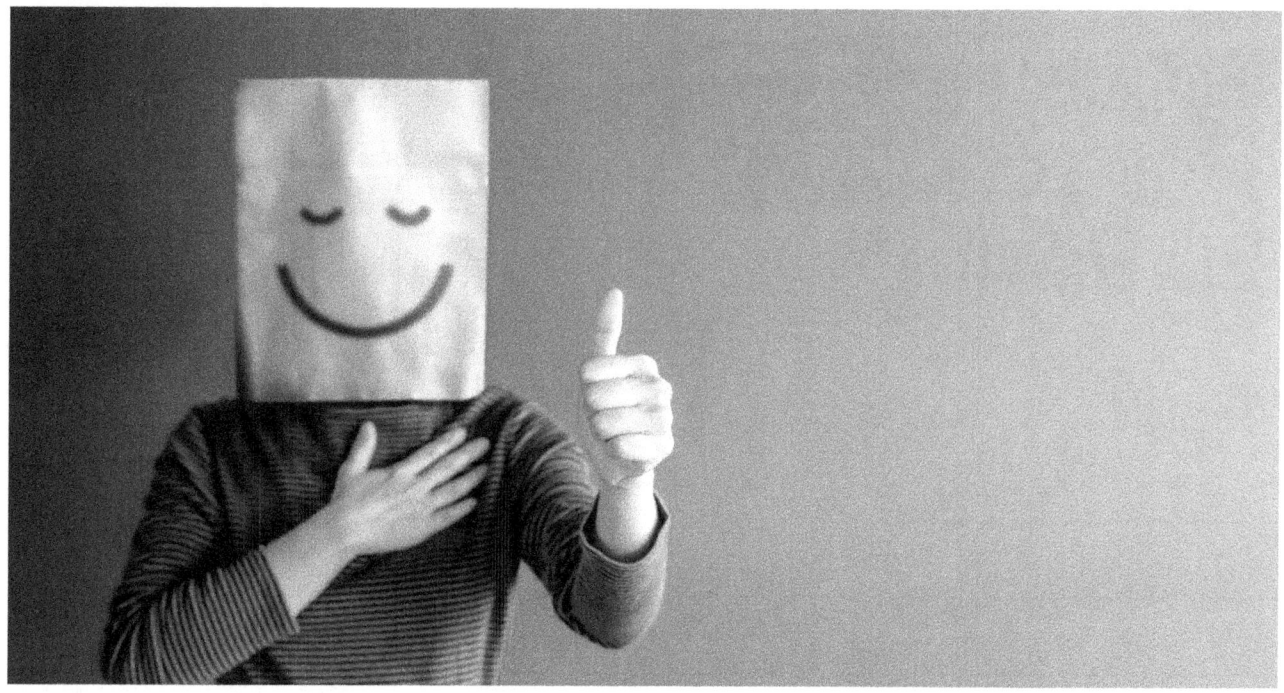

Dear Staff Member,

As one who "straddles the fence," as it were, I understand the challenges and stressors in your workplace. I've worked as an RN in a demanding unit far too long to forget what it's like.

And I understand the patient's point of view. I've passed the twenty-year mark, living with severe chronic pain, and seeking help from medical professionals.

I've lived both lives.

May I thank you on behalf of every patient who comes through your doors this month?

Thank you for every smile, every gentle, human touch. And for calling me by name.

Thank you for reminding us we're not alone in this ever-darkening world of never-ending pain.

Thank you for listening to our concerns and hearing the fear and doubts behind it all. Thank you for listening and attempting to understand.

Thank you for your warmth and kindness, especially when we don't "deserve" it.

Thank you for going the extra mile to ensure consistent care, and to explain important things to me.

With appreciation,
Kristin

Video Clip: How You Treat People Is Who You Are!

(scan the QR code to view the video on YouTube, or transcribe the link—take care, as this link *is* case sensitive)

https://www.youtube.com/watch?v=mTsvSAItPqA

Thoughts:

___
___
___
___
___
___
___
___
___
___
___

Good Examples

Who have you noticed exemplifies superior customer care, implementing strategies we discussed today?

_____

_____

How might you express thanks to that coworker?

_____

_____

How might you model your own interactions with patients after the coworker(s) you admire?

_____

_____

_____

Is there an employee--in any department--who has earned a kind compliment from you, to administration? When and how will you make this known?

_____

_____

_____

You've walked *A Mile In My Shoes*
All that remains is the *Evaluation*

**If you found this training helpful,
your director *needs* to know.**

**If you found this training wanting,
your director *needs* to know.**

Your time and attention to honestly express your feedback is greatly appreciated. The quick circle-your-answer evaluation will take <u>*less than 60 seconds*</u>*. Turn the page!*

Invitation:

Please consider emailing me to let me know how this training helped (or didn't help) your day-to-day challenges at the clinic. I'd love to hear about your experiences as you apply the Three Tools (Strategies)—and how your efforts pay off for your patients and the difference your efforts make for your own job satisfaction and mood.

Don't be shy! I genuinely want to hear from you.

Kristin@KristinHolt.com
(Note: Kristin is spelled without e's)

TRAINING EVALUATION FORM

carefully tear out & give to administrator   **Date:** _____

Name: (optional) _____

Rate the following - ABOUT THE TRAINING CONTENT - on a scale from 1 to 5, where 1 is poor and 5 is excellent:

	POOR				EXCELLENT
The content is helpful and relates to me in my role in this clinic.	1	2	3	4	5
The training content encouraged me to reflect upon my own customer service.	1	2	3	4	5
The training content motivated me to increase my awareness of and performance in customer service.	1	2	3	4	5
The training's use of lecture, videos, self-discovery and discussion was a helpful blend of learning methods.	1	2	3	4	5
This participant's book is helpful.	1	2	3	4	5
I learned something new.	1	2	3	4	5
"Leave Your Stuff At The Door" is an important tool, and applicable to the subject (Walk A Mile In My Shoes)	1	2	3	4	5
"Compassion" is an important tool, and applicable to the subject (Walk A Mile In My Shoes)	1	2	3	4	5
"Kindness" is an important tool, and applicable to the subject (Walk A Mile In My Shoes)	1	2	3	4	5

***The time allotted for this training (60 minutes) was (*circle one*):

just right   inadequate   too much

Evaluation Continues (on back)
Room for Additional Feedback (on back)

Today's trainer's name: _____

Rate the following - ABOUT THE *TRAINER* - on a scale from 1 to 5, where 1 is poor and 5 is excellent:

POOR--------------EXCELLENT

The trainer's volume and enunciation allowed me to hear the presentation.	1	2	3	4	5
The trainer was well-prepared.	1	2	3	4	5
The trainer treated me with courtesy.	1	2	3	4	5
The trainer was qualified to speak on the subject.	1	2	3	4	5

Anything missing from this training?

_____

Additional Feedback:

_____

_____

_____

_____

_____

_____

_____

_____

Appendix A
Twenty-four Pain Lessons

Pain Lesson #24
"We do survive every moment, after all, except the last one."
~ John Updike

Pain Lesson #22
I have learned more from pain than I could've ever learned from pleasure.
- Unknown

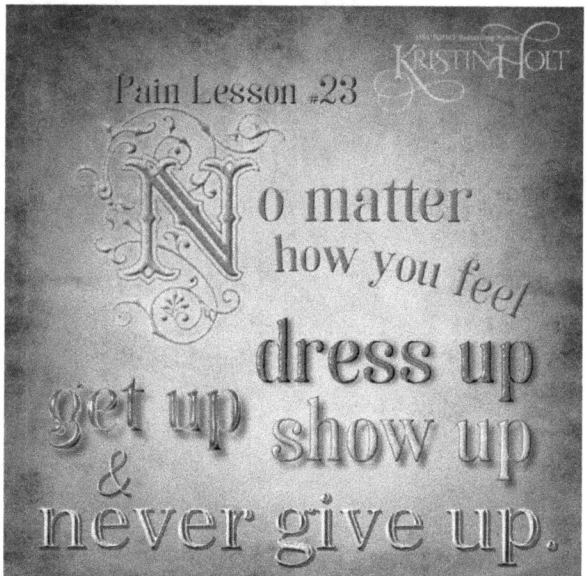

Pain Lesson #23
No matter how you feel dress up get up show up & never give up.

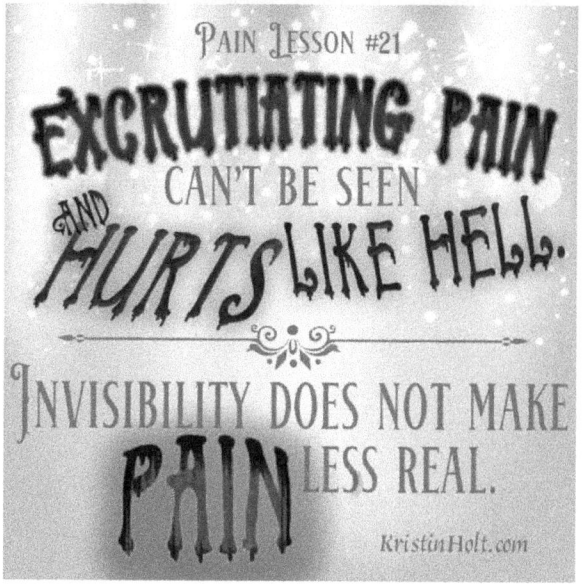

Pain Lesson #21
Excruciating pain can't be seen and hurts like hell. Invisibility does not make pain less real.

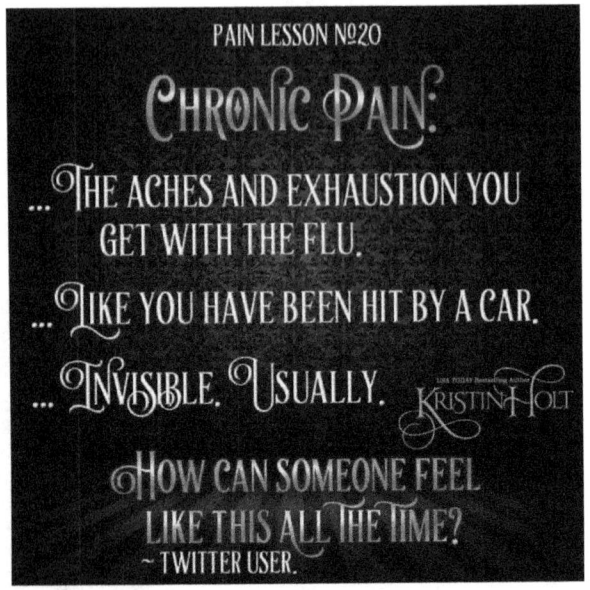
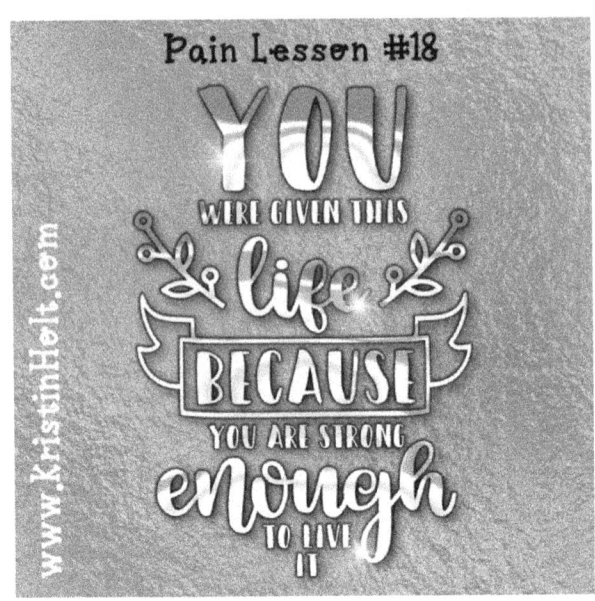
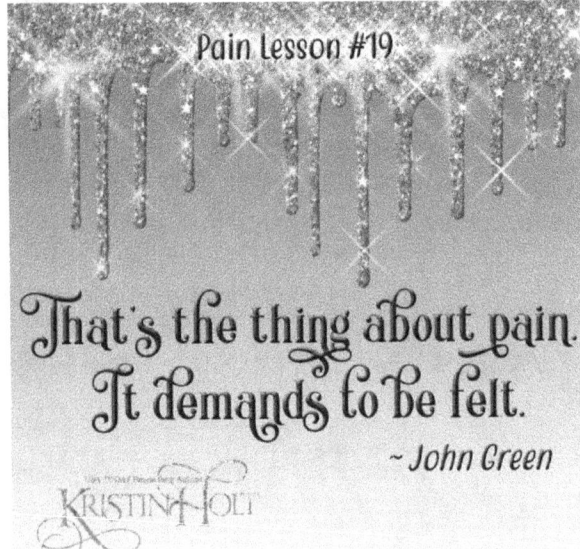
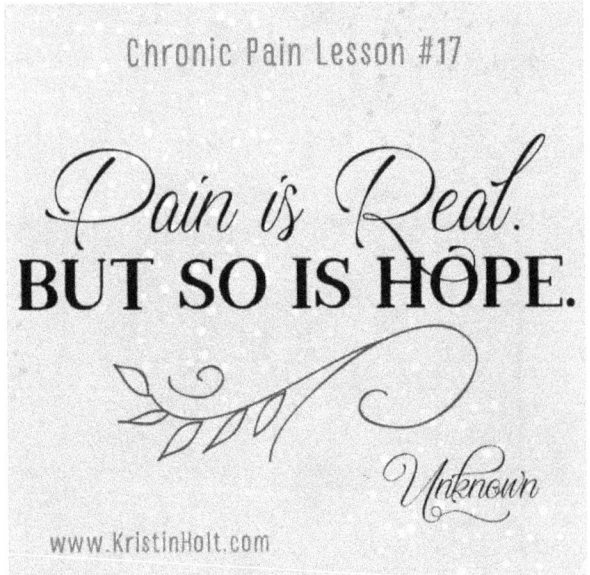

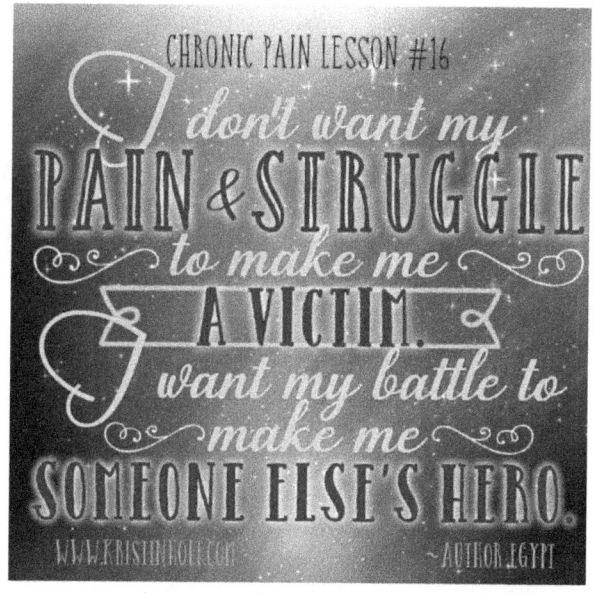
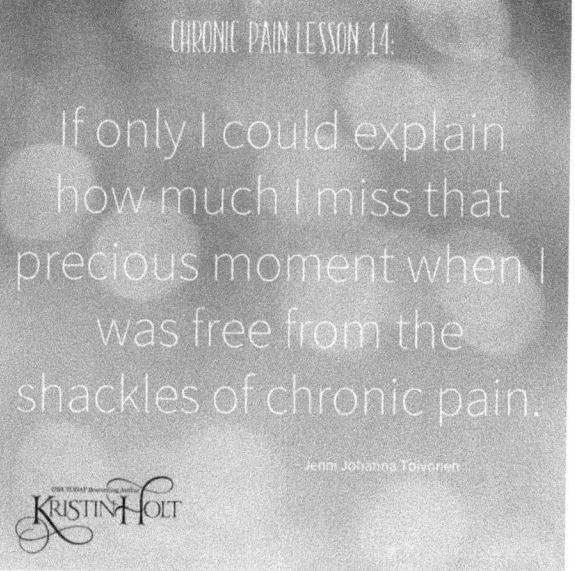

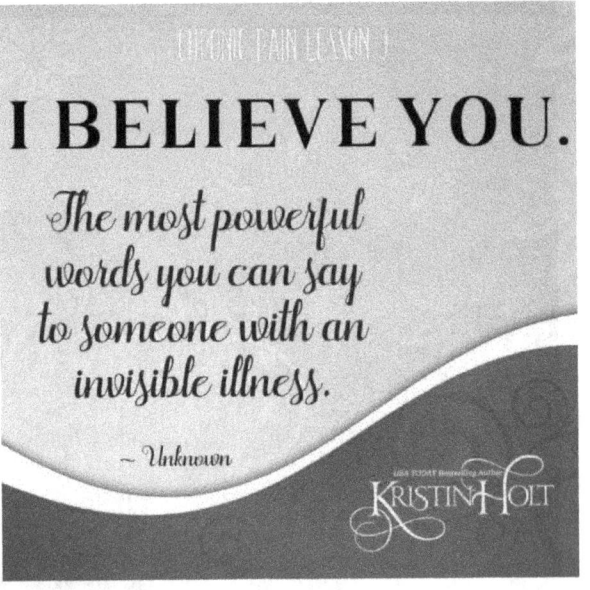

CHRONIC PAIN LESSON 8:

My pain isn't who I am, but it controls what I can do, and in this world, what you can do is a huge measure of who you are.

— LIFEINSLOWMOTIONBLOG.COM

CHRONIC PAIN LESSON 6:
"How are you?"

"I'm really not OK but I don't want to be the reason you're no longer smiling. I don't want to bring sadness to your day or burden you with the heavy load I am carrying. So I say I'm fine, because I don't want you to feel even a fraction of the hurt I do."

— THE MIGHTY (ERIN MIGDOL, STAFF WRITER)

CHRONIC PAIN LESSON 7:

The Mayday Fund estimates 70 million Americans suffer with chronic pain. That's 30.7% of the population.
Women = 34.3%,
Men = 26.7%.

— WIKIPEDIA: CHRONIC PAIN

CHRONIC PAIN LESSON 5:
"I'm fine" doesn't really mean "I'm fine."

I don't really feel like telling you the truth. I am not fine. I haven't been fine for an awfully long time. I just get tired of saying what is really going on.

— THE MIGHTY (ERIN MIGDOL, STAFF WRITER)

CHRONIC PAIN LESSON 4:

"My doctors, who are not cavalier with prescriptions, give me this medication because I have earned their trust. And yet, with mounting government and public pressure, my doctors' hands are becoming tied. They apologetically explain to me why they are required to make the medication even harder for me to get, against their own medical judgment. If the day ever comes when they aren't allowed to prescribe Percocet to me at all, it may well be the end of the minimal quality of life I fight so hard to achieve."

CHRONIC PAIN LESSON 3:

"The addiction crisis is terrifying, and many people don't comprehend opioid use. When I first started taking pain medication, I remember a family member saying, 'Diane, you're going to become an addict!' We need to help people understand that taking pain medicine to maximize one's ability to be productive and to sustain enriching relationships is very different than the disease of addiction, which limits one's ability to contribute to society and maintain healthy habits."

~ DIANE BOURDUE

CHRONIC PAIN LESSON 2:

"You just do it. You force yourself to get up. You force yourself to put one foot before the other and you refuse to let it get you down. You fight. You cry. Then you go about the business of living. That's how I've done it. There is no other way."

— Kristin Holt, USA TODAY Bestselling Author

CHRONIC PAIN LESSON 1:

"You can't get much done in life if you only work on the days when you feel good."

~ JERRY WEST

www.ingramcontent.com/pod-product-compliance
Lightning Source LLC
Chambersburg PA
CBHW080941040426
42444CB00015B/3396